Trends in Memory Development Research

Contributions to Human Development

Vol. 9

Series Editor
John A. Meacham, Buffalo, N.Y.

KARGER

S. Karger · Basel · München · Paris · London · New York · Tokyo · Sydney

Trends in Memory Development Research

Volume Editor
Michelene T.H. Chi, Pittsburgh, Pa.

10 figures and 4 tables, 1983

KARGER

S. Karger · Basel · München · Paris · London · New York · Tokyo · Sydney

Contributions to Human Development

National Library of Medicine, Cataloging in Publication
Trends in memory development research/
volume editor, Michelene T.H. Chi – Basel: Karger, 1983.
(Contributions to human development; v. 9)
Consists of extensively revised papers from a symposium held during the 1981 meeting of the Society for Research in Child Development in Boston.
1. Memory – congresses I. Chi, Michelene T.H. II. Society for Research in Child Development III. Series
W1 C0778s v. 9 [BF 371 T794]
ISBN 3-8055-3661-5

Printed in Switzerland by Boehm-Hutter AG, Reinach BL
ISBN 3-8055-3661-5

Contents

Acknowledgement

Acknowledgement is made for permission to reprint the following material:

Adapted from P.A. Ornstein, M.J. Naus, C. Liberty, Rehearsal and organizational processes in children's memory. Child Development *46:* 818–830. Copyright 1975 by the Society for Research in Child Development. Reprinted by permission of the publisher.

Adapted from P.A. Ornstein, M.J. Naus, B.P. Stone, Rehearsal training and developmental differences in memory. Developmental Psychology *13:* 15–24. Copyright 1977 by the American Psychological Association. Reprinted by permission of the publisher and author.

From C. Liberty, P.A. Ornstein, Age differences in organization and recall: The effects of training in categorization. Journal of Experimental Child Psychology *15:* 169–186. Copyright 1973 by the Academic Press. Reprinted by permission of the publisher.

From D. Klahr, Rages over stages. The Behavioral and Brain Sciences *2:* 191–192. Copyright 1978 by the Cambridge University Press. Reprinted by permission of the publisher.

From H.M. Wellman, J. Collins, G. Gleiberman, Understanding the combination of memory variables: Developing conceptions of memory limitations. Child Development *52:* 1313–1317. Copyright 1981 by the Society for Research in Child Development. Reprinted by permission of the publisher.

To
John Flavell

Preface

At the 1971 meeting of the Society for Research in Child Development (SRCD) in Minneapolis, *John Flavell* organized a landmark symposium entitled 'What is Memory Development the Development of?' That symposium has undoubtedly been an important motivation for the flourishing field of memory development research over the last decade, particularly since the papers from the symposium were made widely available through publication in the journal *Human Development* in 1971. Those symposium papers were personally inspiring, and led me to do my dissertation on what effect changing knowledge has on age-related memory improvements. Memory span, the number of items in a list which can be remembered after a short time, increases with age. I found that this increase is related, at least in part, to increasing familiarity with typical list items due to the experience which comes with age. This relationship of existing knowledge to remembering is a question which many have pursued over the past decade and will undoubtedly continue to pursue in the future, and is a major theme of this volume.

My reflections upon the contribution of that symposium and on the past decade of research led me to consider, in particular, what questions are now being asked in contemporary memory development research. Therefore, a symposium was organized for the 1981 meeting of SRCD in Boston, in honor of the tenth anniversary of the original symposium, to address the current issues in memory development research. Since then, the papers from the symposium have been extensively revised to incorporate comments and suggestions arising during the symposium, as well as the results of recent investigations which have become available since then. In addition to four chapters on current research topics, the final two discussion chapters provide a general overview of the past decade and a look at the future. *Gary Olson* compares and contrasts the current set with those from a decade ago, and *Tom Trabasso* anticipates what the future of memory research might be like.

In 1971, the papers were dominated by a single theme: the role of mnemonic strategies, which are methods that one can use to aid remembering. This was particularly evident in three of the papers. *John Belmont* and *Earl Butterfield* argued that the development of short-term memory involves basically increased and more flexible use of spontaneous rehearsal; that is, repeating the items to be remembered over and over. *John Hagen* pointed out that verbal labeling, attaching names to nonverbal stimuli such as pictures of animals, can be used in conjunction with rehearsal, and discussed the general problem of how children might learn mnemonic strategies. Finally, *Marshall Haith* discussed how young children's lesser ability to remember multiple stimuli presented in a brief visual display might be related to a deficiency in strategies to focus attention selectively on individual parts of the display. In the present volume, the paper by *Mary Naus* and *Peter Ornstein* continues the analysis of the development of memory strategies, but with an emphasis that reflects the theme of the present volume. They consider the extent to which the use of strategies is linked to the child's growing knowledge base.

A second, much less prominent topic in the 1971 symposium was the role of knowledge about storage and retrieval processes. The child, in addition to acquiring memory strategies, will also become more aware and more knowledgeable about what strategies are available, when to use them, and what they can accomplish. It was *John Flavell*, in his discussion, who pointed out the importance of knowledge of one's own memory abilities and who named this knowledge metamemory. *John Hagen* also alluded to metamemory when he argued that, with experience, children discover that their behavior determines how well they remember and thus they are motivated to learn and perfect strategies. Since then, research on metamemory and the more general topic of metacognition, knowledge of all of one's cognitive abilities, has become quite popular. In this volume, *Henry Wellman* summarizes the state of the art in metamemory research, tactfully points out the problems and shortcomings that have been encountered, and offers some insights about how future research should proceed.

David Corsini stressed a third aspect of children's memory abilities, changes in the way they represent the external world in memory. In particular, very young children may be able to remember the world only in terms of what actions they can perform on it, an enactive representation. Somewhat older children can use an iconic representation and remember visual scenes. At a still later age, children develop the ability to attach verbal or conceptual labels to the world and remember it through symbolic representation. In this volume, *Katherine Nelson, Robyn Fivush, Judith Hudson*, and *Joan Lucariello* are also concerned about the issue of representation. However, instead of postulating representational changes with development, they assume that one basic form of representation can be used to characterize both children's and adults' knowledge. Representational abilities such as those discussed by *Corsini* are still necessary before this basic representation can be used, however. The formalism they have chosen is the script, which can describe the structure and use of both children's and adults' knowledge relating to stereotyped sequences of events, such as eating in a restaurant. They examine how children acquire and use such script knowledge and how the content of their scripts affects what they remember.

As I have noted, the role of the knowledge base is a primary theme of this volume. That was not true of the previous symposium; however, the role of knowledge was certainly not ignored. For example, *Corsini* recognized that 'what is coded by the human organism... is determined by the existing cognitive store' (p. 231) and that memory development is 'the development of a general information base' (p. 234). Metamnemonic knowledge is also part of the knowledge base, and its importance was alluded to by both *John Flavell* and *John Hagen*. *Flavell* not only discussed knowledge about memory processes, but also noted that 'all that knowledge... shape(s) what and how we learn and remember' (p. 273).

In some sense, knowledge is the topic of all the chapters in this volume: *Naus and Ornstein* consider the relationship of knowledge to the use of strategies; *Wellman* discussed knowledge about memory processes; *Nelson* et al. describe the content of script knowledge. However, only in the last paper, written by *Ernest Rees* and myself, is development viewed explicitly as the acquisition of new knowledge, the restructuring of existing knowledge, and the integration of new and existing knowledge. Since knowledge acquisition and restructuring are the fundamental processes of learning, it may be that, aside from neurological development in the very early years, development is entirely learning. If this is so, then, in a sense, development is a process that continues throughout adulthood, and thus we anticipate that possible parallels between child development and adult acquisition of expertise will be a fruitful arena of future research.

This volume will be of potential interest not only to specialists in child development, but also to a much wider audience. For instance, as *Gary Olson* points out in his discussion, educators can certainly benefit from an increased understanding of the changing state of children's memories as they pass through school. In addition, education certainly does not stop when adulthood is reached. In industry and the military, for instance, it is vitally important to teach complex, sophisticated skills as efficiently as possible. The same is true in medical schools where vast amounts of knowledge must be acquired in a reasonable span of time. Assuming that the same basic learning processes and memory structures that are present during child development are present in the adult, but presumably in a much more complicated form, the study of child development should shed light on the teaching and acquisition of adult skills. Also, the research reported here should have implications for people who are trying to teach skills and knowledge to individuals with low aptitude, since they have deficiencies that children characteristically exhibit.

Because it is clear from these chapters that the question 'What is memory development the development of?' is still only partly answered, I hope this volume will stimulate many more exciting investigations of memory development and learning, as well as generate many more thesis topics. I gratefully acknowledge the help of *Ernest Rees* in the various phases of editing this volume, and the help of *Polly Bitzer* in typing all the manuscripts into their final forms. Preparation of this volume was supported by the Learning Research and Development Center, which is funded in part by the National Institute of Education. My support from the Spencer Foundation as a National Academy of Education Fellow is also acknowledged with gratitude.

Micki Chi

Contr. hum. Dev., vol. 9, pp. 1–30 (Karger, Basel 1983)

Development of Memory Strategies: Analysis, Questions, and Issues

Mary J. Naus, Peter A. Ornstein[1]

Haverford College, Haverford, Pa.; University of North Carolina at Chapel Hill, Chapel Hill, N.C., USA

The years since *Flavell's* [1971] landmark symposium 'What is memory development the development of?' have witnessed continually growing interest in memory development in children. In this paper, we will focus on an aspect of this flourishing research tradition that was well-represented at that symposium: skilled mnemonic techniques. After characterizing our perception of the state of the art in 1971, we will briefly analyze research investigating the development of memory strategies in the last decade, using our own work [*Ornstein and Naus,* 1978; *Ornstein and Corsale,* 1979a] as an example. Much has been learned about children's deployment of memory techniques, but there are nonetheless a number of unanswered questions that limit our current understanding of the emergence of the skilled use of these procedures. Accordingly, we have selected four interrelated and as yet unanswered questions to guide discussion concerning the direction of future research. Although each of these questions is important from the point of view of a thorough understanding of strategy development in young children, we have selected one issue – the link between strategy development and the child's growing knowledge base in permanent memory – as most critical and will present some new data that are relevant to this problem.

Research on Children's Memory: 1971

A brief survey of the papers presented at the 1971 symposium illustrates the state of the art in the study of memory development in preschool

[1] This work was supported in part by Grant HD 08459 from the National Institute of Child Health and Human Development.

and elementary school children during the late 1960s and early 1970s. In the first of four major presentations, *Corsini* [1971] called attention to a number of important factors, such as the form of the initial representation of to-be-remembered materials and the subject's perception of task demands, that affect the level of memory performance. In the second paper, *Haith* [1971] focused on visual sensory memory, suggesting that there are minimal age-related changes in the 'hardware' of the memory system, in contrast to developmentally sensitive subject-controlled processes. In the final two papers, *Belmont and Butterfield* [1971] and *Hagen* [1971] discussed research on the development of verbal mnemonic strategies in short-term memory. *Belmont and Butterfield* [1971] used a pause-time procedure to draw inferences about age-related changes in the use of strategies as a function of task requirements, chronological age, and mental status. In the context of a probe recall task, *Hagen* [1971] compared the serial position function of spontaneous and instructed verbal labelers so as to draw inferences about developmental changes in the use of labeling as a deliberate strategy.

A number of general comments describing the state of the field at this time can be made on the basis of these four papers. First, as was the case with memory research in general, all authors seemed to assume implicitly an information processing orientation with an informal focus on multistore models [*Atkinson and Shiffrin,* 1968, 1971]. The emphasis was on the sensory and short-term components of the memory system and, although the role of memory strategies in the encoding and storage of information in long-term memory was acknowledged, none of the symposium papers dealt explicitly with the development of general knowledge in permanent memory. Second, although one of the major themes of the symposium was that of the development of verbal memory strategies, the methodologies used to study these techniques, by and large, did not allow direct observation of them. Rather, age-related changes in the implementation of particular memory strategies were inferred on the basis of presumably correlated response measures. Disadvantages associated with this inferential approach, as opposed to the direct observation of memory strategies, are discussed by *Ornstein and Naus* [1978]. Third, a prevalent explanatory concept invoked at the symposium to account for age-related changes in memory strategy usage was *Flavell's* [1970] production deficiency notion. However, because the production deficiency concept is primarily descriptive, calling attention to discrepancies between available knowledge and the spontaneous use of this information in a strategic sense, the research reported at the symposium did not really concern itself with the circumstances under which, or the mechanisms by which, sophisticated mnemonic strategy usage emerges. Other difficulties with the concept have been discussed by *Paris* [1978a].

Research on the Development of Memory Strategies: 1971–1981

A number of the views expressed at the *Flavell* [1971] symposium set the stage for research on strategy development during the 1970s. The information processing approach continued to dominate the field, albeit with a strong movement away from the multistore memory framework and with considerable interest in alternative memory metaphors [*Bransford* et al. 1977; *Brown,* 1975; *Craik and Lockhart,* 1972; *Naus and Halasz*, 1979; *Naus* et. al., 1978; *Ornstein and Corsale,* 1979b; *Paris,* 1978b]. In addition, in at least some quarters, research continued to focus on the development of verbal memory strategies such as rehearsal and organization. However, during this decade, tasks that permitted the direct observation of these memory strategies were employed. The investigation of the development of rehearsal strategies was advanced by the application of *Rundus'* [1971] and *Rundus and Atkinson's* [1970] overt rehearsal procedure [*Ornstein and Naus,* 1978], and the study of the development of organizational strategies was aided by the use of variations of *Mandler's* [1967] sorting procedure [*Ornstein and Corsale,* 1979a]. Both of these methodologies permit a focus upon the dynamics by which particular mnemonic strategies operate and develop, rather than the purely mediational aspects of strategy usage that were emphasized in the previous decade. Our work on the development of verbal rehearsal and organization in elementary school age children provides a clear example of this approach.

Rehearsal Strategies

Our studies of verbal rehearsal have used variations of the overt rehearsal procedure with children of various ages. In addition to describing age-related differences in children's rehearsal techniques, we have established a direct, causal relationship between developmental changes in rehearsal and recall performance, and we have begun to address theoretical questions such as how age-related changes in rehearsal strategies affect memory encoding, storage, and retrieval [*Ornstein and Naus,* 1978].

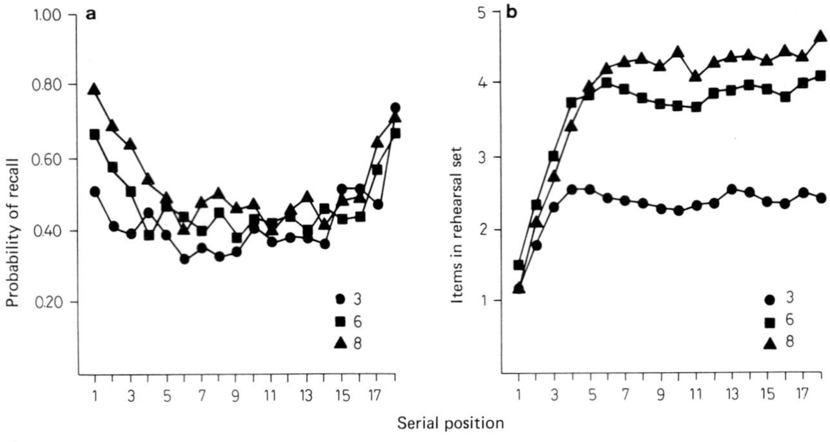

Fig. 1. Mean proportion of unrelated items recalled (*a*) and mean number of different items in each rehearsal set (*b*) as a function of serial position for third-, sixth-, and eighth-grade subjects [from *Ornstein* et al., 1975].

In an initial experiment, *Ornstein* et al. [1975; experiment I] asked third, sixth, and eighth graders to overtly rehearse 18 unrelated items in a free recall task. The subjects were required to rehearse aloud as each list item was presented and then to recall the words in any order. As can be seen in figure 1a, recall performance, especially that of the initial items, improved with age. Further, an analysis of the children's rehearsal 'sets', the rehearsal associated with the presentation of each new item, revealed parallel age-related changes. More specifically, the third graders tended to repeat only one or two different items together as each new word was presented ('passive rehearsal'), whereas the older children practiced each newly presented word along with several previously displayed list items ('active rehearsal'). These data, averaged over all children at each grade, are displayed in figure 1b, and indicate that there are substantial age changes in rehearsal activity, as measured by the number of different or unique items that are rehearsed together.

Additional support for a direct relationship between rehearsal activity and recall performance was obtained in a series of training studies in which the rehearsal strategies of both younger and older children were manipulated directly, resulting in corresponding changes in recall performance [*Naus* et al., 1977a; *Ornstein* et al., 1977b]. *Ornstein* et al. [1977b], for example, examined a number of rehearsal strategies that differed in terms of rehearsal set content. Second and sixth graders studied a list of 18 unrelat-

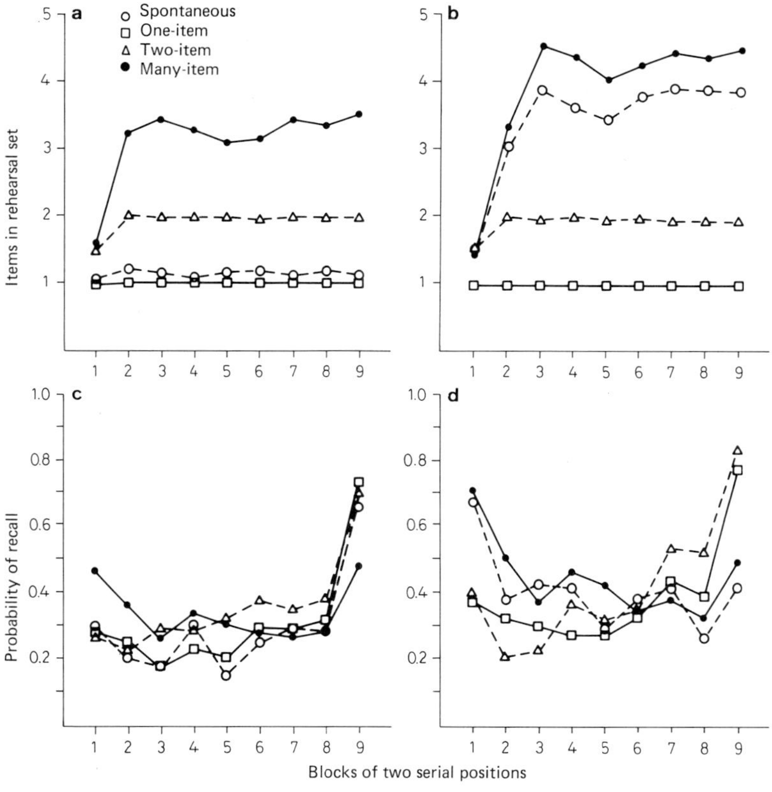

Fig. 2. Mean number of different items per rehearsal set and mean proportion of items recalled as a function of serial position for second (*a, c*) and sixth-grade (*b, d*) subjects under different instructional conditions [from *Ornstein* et al., 1977b].

ed words according to one of several suggested techniques: a one-item strategy in which only the currently presented word was rehearsed (passive rehearsal), a two-item strategy in which the currently presented word was rehearsed with the previously displayed item, or a many-item strategy in which an attempt was made to rehearse together several different items (active rehearsal). At each age level, the performance of these three groups was compared to a spontaneous rehearsal group which did not receive any particular rehearsal instructions.

The results of this study (fig. 2) indicate that the recall of initial list items varied as a function of level of rehearsal activity. Second graders spontaneously rehearsed in a fashion similar to those subjects in the one-

and two-item instructed conditions, but they could follow a many-item strategy when so instructed. Further, as indicated in figure 2, recall performance varied as a function of rehearsal technique, with the serial position curves of the second-grade spontaneous, one-, and two-item subjects showing a flat primacy portion. In contrast, the primacy portion of the curve was substantially elevated for second graders using a many-item strategy. Sixth graders spontaneously rehearsed in a manner that was similar to the many-item instructed subjects, and could easily follow the one- and two-item instructions. Those rehearsing according to the many-item strategy or who were rehearsing spontaneously demonstrated a substantial primacy effect, whereas the primacy effect was eliminated from the sixth graders in the two passive rehearsal training conditions. This experiment clearly established a direct functional relationship between the type of rehearsal strategy used and recall performance.

Other studies in our research program have explored the mechanisms by which active rehearsal facilitates the recall of older children. For example, *Naus* et al. [1977b] addressed the question of whether active rehearsal affects primarily the storage or retrieval of information in permanent memory. Our results suggested that differences in rehearsal activity influence the ease of item retrieval from long-term memory, but that these effects are mediated by differences in the stored representation of the items. *Ornstein* et al. [1977a] confirmed suggestions made by *Ornstein* et al. [1975; experiment II] that active rehearsal may operate by generating associative connections among the to-be-remembered items. Consistent with this notion, the data also suggested that the effects of active rehearsal are minimized when the to-be-remembered items contain a highly salient organizational structure. Further, *Stone* et al. [1977] verified the importance of active rehearsal in establishing an organizational plan during learning, and also eliminated an alternative point of view concerning the mechanism by which active rehearsal influences recall. Specifically, the data of *Stone* et al. [1977] suggest that practice at retrieving information during rehearsal is not responsible for the facilitative effects of active rehearsal [see *Ornstein and Naus,* 1978, for a more detailed review of this work].

Organizational Strategies

Similar progress has also been made, by the use of direct observational procedures, in understanding the role of organizational strategies in the development of children's memory [*Ornstein and Corsale,* 1979b]. As is the case with the work investigating rehearsal, the research on children's

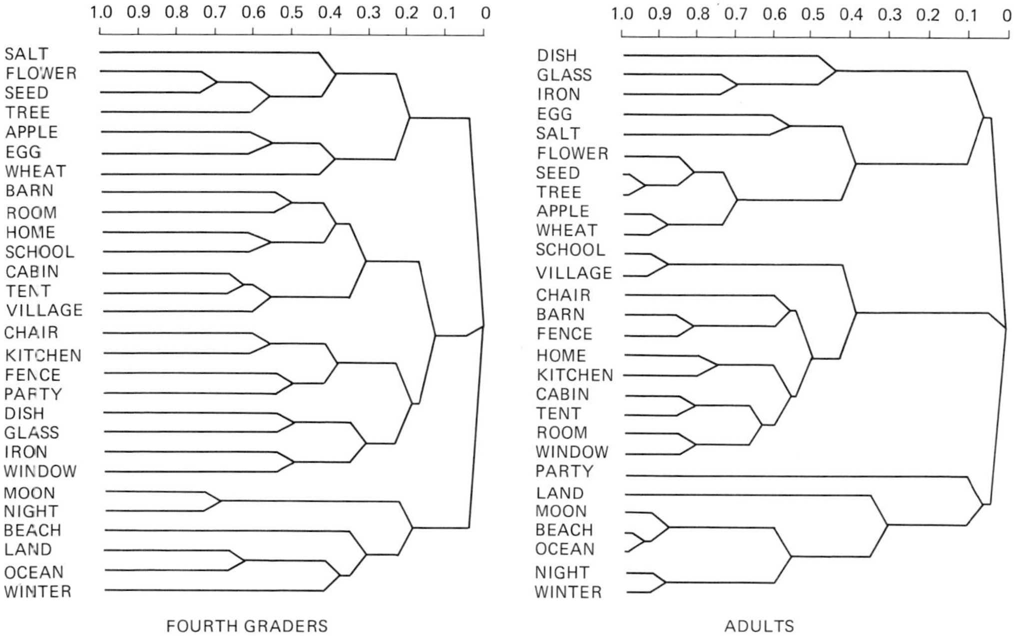

Fig. 3. Hierarchical clustering solutions, based on intersubject sorting agreement, for fourth graders and adults given unrelated items [from *Liberty and Ornstein*, 1973].

organizational strategies suggests that young children engage in less systematic attempts at organizing than do older children when recall is explicitly requested.

Liberty and Ornstein [1973] observed differences in sorting or input organization, as well as in recall, when fourth graders and college-age subjects were presented with 28 unrelated items for alternating sort/recall trials. Free-sorting subjects were instructed to sort items together on any basis, such that the groups formed would facilitate recall; by contrast, other subjects were provided with specific sorting patterns to 'learn'. Figure 3 presents the data for the free-sorting subjects in the form of tree structure diagrams resulting from the application of hierarchical clustering procedures [*Johnson,* 1967; *Ornstein and Corsale,* 1979b]. The axis in figure 3 represents the proportion of subjects who sorted various groups of items together. Thus, examination of the left panel indicates that approximately 70% of the fourth graders sorted the words *flower* and *seed* together. As can be seen, the free sorting fourth graders tended to form seemingly random, nonsemantically constrained groups, whereas the adults generated highly organized groupings based upon the meanings of the items. In addition, the proportion of subjects grouping particular clusters of items together is higher for the adults than the children, suggesting that the sorting patterns of the fourth graders were relatively idiosyncratic, whereas those of the adults were consistent with each other.

The lower degree of semantic organization present in the young children's sorts was reflected in the poorer recall of these subjects. Further, those constrained fourth graders who learned the sorting patterns generated by adults recalled more items than other children required to group items according to patterns developed by other fourth graders. Similarly, the adults who were constrained to the grouping patterns of fourth graders exhibited lower recall scores than those learning the sorts of other adults. These findings indicate that the semantic characteristics of the groupings formed prior to recall are related directly to recall success.

Although *Liberty and Ornstein's* [1973] free sorting fourth graders did not make use of the underlying semantic relationships in the formation of their sorting patterns, subsequent questioning indicated that they were nonetheless aware of these relationships. In fact, when asked to form groups of items 'that go together', their sorting patterns were as highly constrained as those of the adults. This finding, implying that elementary-school-age children may have knowledge of semantic relations available in the to-be-remembered material but do not use this information spontaneously in the service of a memory goal, was explored in a subsequent series of experiments conducted by *Bjorklund* et al. [1977]. Extending the findings of *Liberty and Ornstein* [1973], *Bjorklund* et al. [1977] showed that requiring third and fifth graders to sort according to the patterns generated by adults could result in enhanced recall. However, in order for the constrained sorting procedure to be effective with the third graders, additional instructions concerning the semantic nature of the adult categories were required [*Bjorklund* et al., 1977; experiment II]. Interestingly, it was found [*Bjorklund* et al., 1977; experiment III] that these instructions alone, without the requirement of physical sorting in adult-determined patterns, were sufficient to lead to improved recall.

Other experiments in our laboratory have extended these demonstrations that young children do not necessarily organize spontaneously when instructed to remember relatively impoverished stimulus materials, but have the underlying knowledge to support organizational activities. *Corsale and Ornstein* [1980], for example, have shown that recall performance will vary as a function of the extent to which the items are grouped semantically, regardless of whether a recall test is expected. Thus, third graders presented with a list of unrelated items and instructed to form meaningful groups recall more on an unexpected incidental memory test than those doing spontaneous sorts in preparation for recall. Further, recent data have shown that there are conditions of list structure under which young children may organize spontaneously in the service of memory goals. Thus, for example, with categorically related items, third graders will often sort spontaneously in a meaningful fashion [*Corsale,* 1978], and these sorting experiences can provide conditions conducive to the induction of task appropriate organizational strategies with unrelated materials [*Best and Ornstein,* 1979].

Summary

The direct observational procedures used to study the development of rehearsal and organizational strategies have permitted major advances in our understanding of mnemonic techniques. Going beyond the inferential procedures which characterized earlier research [*Hagen,* 1971; *Belmont and Butterfield,* 1971], it has been possible to conduct detailed analyses of these strategies, the conditions under which they are utilized, and to some extent the mechanisms by which they operate. It seems clear that during the elementary school years children gain facility in the implementation of a broad range of mnemonic skills and that this strategic growth involves subtle changes in the nature and application of these techniques. Further, and perhaps more importantly, this detailed understanding of memory strategies provides the necessary background for addressing a number of major issues in memory development which have yet to be adequately explored.

Unanswered Questions

We have identified four major classes of issues that may set the stage for research on the operation of memory strategies in the 1980s. First, relatively little is known about those factors that influence the emergence of skilled organizational and rehearsal strategies during the later elementary school years. Second, the relationship between children's early mnemonic abilities during the preschool years and the more adult-like skills observed later needs to be determined. Third, attention needs to be directed to the fundamental issues of the very definition of a mnemonic strategy. Finally, the effects of the specific mnemonic context on the use of memory strategies remain to be investigated; research examining strategy development to date can be criticized in that it deals with memory in very limited situations, and does not adequately take into consideration such factors as the child's knowledge of the to-be-remembered materials. The first three of these issues will be discussed briefly below, whereas the fourth will be dealt with in a final section devoted to strategy development in the context of the changing knowledge base in permanent memory.

What Factors Affect the Emergence of Mnemonic Skills?

The literature summarized above suggests that young children often have information available in permanent memory that they do not bring to bear in a strategic sense in the context of a memory task. Yet, by the end of the elementary school years, they are capable of spontaneously utilizing a variety of sophisticated mnemonic techniques. Although the past decade has witnessed major advances in documenting the age-related changes in strategy usage, little progress has been made in addressing the question of why these developmental changes in the way in which stored information is utilized are found.

The concept of metamemory (i.e. children's knowledge about their own memory functioning) was proposed during the 1970s as a possible explanation for strategy development during the elementary school years [*Brown*, 1979; *Flavell and Wellman*, 1977; *Kail*, 1979; *Wellman*, 1977]. Initial investigations of metamemory development focused only on describing children's changing knowledge of the operation of memory, as judged by means of interview techniques [*Kreutzer* et al., 1975]. However, recent work [reviewed by *Kail*, 1979; *Wellman*, 1977] has investigated directly the relationship between metamemory and memory performance across age [*Brown*, 1979; *Levin* et al., 1977; *Miller* et al., 1977; *Stern* et al., 1981; *Wellman and Johnson*, 1979; *Yussen and Levy*, 1975; *Yussen and Paquette*, 1978].

Brown [1979] described a number of alternative conceptions concerning the linkage between metamemory and actual memory performance, but when metamemory is considered an explanatory concept for strategy development, then the adult-like deployment of mnemonic strategies is considered to follow directly from the child's growing awareness of the functioning of his or her own memory and the utility of more effective mnemonic techniques. Unfortunately, however, the relationship between metamemory and actual memory performance has not been consistent, although some development trends in metamemory behavior have been established [see reviews by *Kail*, 1979; *Wellman*, 1977]. Given the absence of even systematic correlations between these two aspects of memory development, it is difficult to consider metamemory as instrumental in the emergence of sophisticated mnemonic techniques.

Although at present specific factors that might be important in the development of mnemonic strategies have not been specified, recent cross-cultural work on literacy [*Cole and Scribner*, 1974; *Luria*, 1976; *Wagner*, 1978] suggests one possible approach to this problem. In general, cross-cultural studies implicate participation in a formal educational setting as being of importance for the development of adult-like memory strategies. A variety of studies has demonstrated that individuals who have been exposed to formal education differ markedly in the use of planful mnemonic strategies from their same-age peers who have not attended school. Thus, skilled strategy usage seems to be associated with participation in formal schooling and related activities [*Sharp* et al., 1979]. However, although school seems important, we currently lack direct evidence concerning the linkage between school activities and cognitive growth.

It is also quite difficult to determine exactly which school experiences are of critical importance for strategic development, especially given that teachers do not in general provide much explicit training in memory skills [*Feurstein*, 1980; *Medlin*, 1978]. It seems likely that certain in-class activities require the use of mental activities that are relevant to remembering and may contribute to the development of adult memory skills. Further, it may be the case that teachers' requests for memorization bring about induction of task-appropriate strategy usage independent of any direct instruction. Consistent with this notion, *Best and Ornstein* [1979] demonstrated that third graders can be induced to use sophisticated mnemonic techniques after exposure to a number of memory 'problems' in a learning set fashion. These findings may be interpreted as suggesting that children can form generalized strategies as a result of repeated exposure in school to activities requiring grouping, classification, and remembering. It seems clear, though, that detailed analysis of classroom activities and their relationship to memory processing should be one research goal for the 1980s.

What Is the Relationship between a Child's Early and Later Memory Abilities?

The research investigating strategy development [*Ornstein and Corsale*, 1979a; *Ornstein and Naus*, 1978] has focused primarily upon the dramatic age-related changes in mnemonic processing which occur during the elementary school years. To what extent is the elementary school child's development of a repertoire of skilled mnemonic strategies paralleled by related achievements during the preschool years? Relatively little attention has been paid to the documentation of the memorization skills of the preschool child or to the critical issue of the relationship between these early skills and those that develop later.

The implication of research concerned with the memory performance of school-aged children, such as that discussed above, would be that preschoolers are inefficient memorizers. In fact, however, the situation appears to be more complicated. Under appropriate conditions, the memory performance of preschool children can be remarkably planful and sophisticated, as we have learned from informal naturalistic studies [*Perlmutter*, 1980], as well as laboratory investigations [*Myers and Perlmutter*, 1978; *Ratner and Myers*, 1980]. In this regard, data collected in our laboratory by *Baker-Ward* [1980] suggest that 3- and 4-year olds clearly can differentiate between memory and play situations in terms of the manner in which they interact with presented objects. The ability of these young children to employ differential activities as a function of instructions suggests that even preschoolers have the beginnings of functional mnemonic strategies. Additional work is clearly required to document the types of mnemonic processes these young children can employ across a variety of different settings.

Given that preschoolers seem capable of some level of strategic activity, at least under some conditions, questions concerning the developmental continuity of strategy usage arise. How do the early memory skills that are being detected under some conditions relate to the skilled use of memory strategies in the later elementary school years? To what extent is there a link between a preschool child's ability to use strategies in some particular context and his or her later ability to apply a fully articulated set of strategies across a variety of domains? Longitudinal research addressing this question would seem to constitute an additional research goal for the 1980s.

What Is a Memory Strategy?

Memory strategies have been considered to be task-appropriate cognitive or behavioral activities that are under the deliberate control of the subject and are employed so as to enhance memory performance. This definition of memory strategies seemed straightforward, particularly when these control processes were contrasted with the structural features of memory in the context of multistore conceptualizations of the memory system [*Atkinson and Shiffrin*, 1968, 1971]. However, empirical findings as well as changes in orientation [*Bransford* et al., 1977; *Craik and Lockhart*, 1972; *Naus and Halasz*, 1979; *Schneider and Shiffrin*, 1977; *Shiffrin and Schneider*, 1977] have complicated the task of identifying these deliberately employed memory skills.

There are at least three interrelated issues that have implications for strategy definition and diagnosis. The first reflects the fact that a variety of non-strategic, more-or-less automatic memory processes (e.g. categorization and the formation of inferences) have been identified and studied [*Hasher and Zacks*, 1979; *Naus and Halasz*, 1979; *Ornstein and Naus*, in press; *Schneider and Shiffrin*, 1977; *Shiffrin and Schneider*, 1977]. These automatic processes would clearly seem to be involved in situations in which incidental memory is tested following various orienting tasks [*Corsale and Ornstein*, 1980; *Hyde and Jenkins*, 1969]. Although at present relatively little is known about the operation of these automatic processes, they do seem to stand in contrast to deliberate strategies in that they are unconscious and unplanned. Automatic processing is thought to be initiated in a non-deliberate fashion without (or with limited) attentional demands, reflecting the effects of environmental stimuli operating upon the contents of permanent semantic memory. The fact that these relatively automatic mnemonic processes may have the same consequences as deliberately employed strategies – and that under some conditions children's incidental memory following semantic tasks is better than their deliberate attempts at memorization [*Corsale and Ornstein*, 1980] – raises obvious definitional issues.

Given the existence of automatic mnemonic processing, the second definitional problem stems from the fact that under some conditions, what would appear to be the operation of a mnemonic strategy may actually reflect an automatic process. Thus, for example, *Lange* [1973, 1978] has argued that much of the category clustering that is observed in the free recall of preadolescent children may not reflect the deliberate deployment of a strategy, as has frequently been assumed, but rather may be automatically determined by the associative structure of the materials. This author suggests that clustering is only observed with preadolescents when the stimulus items have very strong associative connections and that it represents a type of automatic exercise of associative pathways that are already pronounced in the permanent memories of these subjects. A final issue relating to the question of definition is that even when we are certain that we are dealing with deliberate memory strategies, the use of these techniques by elementary-school-age children is very much a function of materials and other aspects of the context [*Corsale*, 1978; *Ornstein and Naus*, in press]. The demonstration of *Corsale* [1978] and *Corsale and Ornstein* [1980] that third graders' meaningful sorting in preparation for recall was mentioned briefly above in the summary of research on organizational strategies and will be dealt with below in the broader context of the effects of the knowledge base upon memory performance.

These findings suggest that a third major research theme for the next decade could profitably involve the investigation of developmental changes in the relationship between deliberately employed memory strategies and automatic mnemonic processes in a variety of different contexts. It would appear that our understanding of the definition of memory strategies may in part be determined by a contrast class of automatic processes.

What Are the Effects of Context on the Development and Utilization of Memory Strategies?

Although it was initially assumed that the implementation of memory strategies was context free, changes in the characteristics of the task can have profound effects upon the expression of these strategies. Variations in the materials to be remembered [*Corsale*, 1978], instructions [*Corsale and Ornstein*, 1980; *Naus* et al., 1977a], and formality of the setting [*Istomina*, 1975] all have been shown to affect children's strategic behavior in memory situations [*Ornstein and Corsale*, 1979b]. To a great extent there is a discrepancy between the young child's knowledge and his or her application of that knowledge in a deliberate sense when the goal is that of remembering. Indeed, this discrepancy may represent one of the most salient features of children's memory performance. But it is also the case, certainly through the elementary school years, that the discrepancy between knowledge and its mnemonic utilization varies considerably as a function of context.

Despite growing awareness of the situational specificity of children's memory performance, our understanding of these context effects and their implications for the broader view of the developing memory system is limited because they have neither been explored systematically nor integrated theoretically. At the empirical level, we do not have, for example, adequate documentation of a progression in strategy implementation from situations that are less demanding (measured in some appropriate manner) to those that are more demanding. The findings of *Corsale* [1978] and *Corsale and Ornstein* [1980] of the spontaneous use of task-appropriate sorting strategies with categorical materials before they appear with unrelated materials is suggestive of such a progression, as is *Baker-Ward's* [1980] observations of what seem to be preschoolers' non-verbal strategies. However, there needs to be detailed study of the environments that call forth strategic behavior to varying degrees, and this requires attention to children's incidental and deliberate memory in a wide variety of settings.

Even granted that it is possible to order the context specificity that is present in children's application of memory strategies, attention at a theoretical level needs to be paid to this pervasive aspect of cognitive development. Does experience with categorically related materials permit the child to induce without instruction certain mnemonic skills, as *Best and Ornstein* [1979] speculate? Can these various findings be incorporated into a systematic model of the development of memory? No such model exists at the present time, although Soviet [*Smirnov*, 1973], constructivist [*Paris*, 1978b], and levels-of-processing [*Craik and Lockhart*, 1972] formulations may pave the way for the construction of a truly developmental model [*Ornstein and Corsale*, 1979b].

It seems clear that a fourth major research theme for the 1980s is that of the study of context effects; it is also the case that this work will relate directly to the three other themes discussed above. Although a number of aspects of the mnemonic context need to be investigated in detail, in our current work we have begun to consider one aspect of the problem, namely the linkage between strategy development and the child's changing knowledge of the to-be-remembered materials. As will be seen, a number of our studies [*Ornstein and Naus*, in press, for a more complete overview] have suggested that the growing knowledge base in permanent memory may contribute to the expression of the increasingly more sophisticated rehearsal and organizational strategies that are used by older children. The next section of this paper examines the critical interface between the child's knowledge and the implementation of memory strategies.

Strategy Development in the Context of the Knowledge Base

As the literature described above suggests, a great deal of attention has been devoted to the study of the linkage between children's developing memory strategies and corresponding changes in their recall performance. It has also recently become apparent that in order to understand more fully the operation and development of these strategies, it is necessary to explore the growing knowledge system in permanent memory. Interestingly, in the last several years [*Chi*, 1977, 1978; *Ornstein and Naus*, in press], there have been a number of demonstrations of the influence of the changing knowledge base on age-related improvements in memory performance, without the mediation of mnemonic strategies. The implication of these demonstrations has been that age-related changes in the knowledge base may alone account for developmental differences in memory performance. It is our view, however, that strategy and knowledge-base effects are not incompatible and that progress in understanding memory development requires simultaneous attention to both strategy and knowledge base changes. We feel that knowledge-base effects are often mediated by mnemonic strategies and that the implementation of these strategies may vary substantially as a function of the child's existing state of knowledge [*Ornstein and Naus*, in press].

Knowledge-Base Demonstrations

Major credit for calling attention to the role of the knowledge base in children's memory development must be given to *Chi* [1977, 1978]. *Chi* [1977], for example, showed that both strategy and knowledge base differences contributed to age-related changes in memory span. Under conditions in which the stimuli were equally familiar for the children and adults, and in which adults were prevented from using sophisticated mnemonic strategies, age differences in memory span performance were almost completely eliminated. In further work, *Chi* [1978] investigated the operation of the knowledge base more thoroughly by asking subjects of different ages to remember the position of chess pieces. The degree of knowledge of the game of chess was varied by comparing chess novices to expert chess players. However, in contrast to previous work with adult subjects [*Chase and Simon*, 1973], the novice players in *Chi's* experiments were adults and the experts were children who averaged 10 years of age. The child experts demonstrated better memory for the legitimate positions of chess pieces than did the adult novice players, whereas the findings were reversed in a test of digit span. These data suggest that, independent of overall proficiency in strategy usage, knowledge per se is of critical importance in memory performance. That the children's memory superiority was restricted to the chess domain in which they were experts indicates the importance of specific knowledge and reduces the possibility of alternate explanations.

In addition to *Chi's* [1977, 1978] studies of nonverbal memory, children's verbal memory skills as a function of knowledge base variables have also been investigated. For example, *Lindberg* [1980] compared third graders and adults on words drawn from standard taxonomic categories and those taken from children's school experiences (e.g. names of school teachers, titles of books, etc.). Children's recall was substantially facilitated with the child-centered materials, reflecting the influence of the knowledge base in verbal memory tasks. Other demonstrations that the knowledge base contributes importantly to memory development have been reported in the studies of stimulus meaningfulness [*Richman* et al., 1976], as well as those carried out within context of levels-of-processing [*Peterson*, 1977; *Weiss* et al., 1977] and Piagetian [*Piaget and Inhelder*, 1973] points of view.

Although there are methodological problems with some of these studies [*Ornstein and Naus*, in press, provide a critique], it is clear that the state of knowledge in permanent memory seriously affects memory performance and that changes in knowledge with age contribute to corresponding improvements in memory. On the other hand, our understanding of the influence of the knowledge base is rather limited; in fact, we are not much beyond the level of demonstrations of correlations between measures of knowledge (however defined) and memory performance. For example, with *Chi's* work on chess, the correlation between an individual's status (e.g. expert versus novice) and recall does not constitute an explanation of how such differences arise. We do not have any information concerning how age differences in the information stored in permanent memory mediate differences in the encoding, storage, or retrieval of information.

To begin to understand the critical link between what is stored in permanent memory and the ability to remember currently presented information, it is necessary to study jointly the effects of the knowledge base and mnemonic strategies. Ideally, the concurrent investigation of mnemonic processes and knowledge base changes would entail (a) the detailed specification of development changes in selected knowledge domains, and (b) the assessment of mnemonic strategy usage in tasks involving materials drawn from these domains, as a function of both knowledge development and age. Unfortunately at present, such investigations have not been reported in the developmental literature. However, a number of recently completed studies concerning strategy usage with varying sets of stimulus materials permit us to make initial inferences concerning the strategy/knowledge base interaction.

Rehearsal Strategies

Ornstein and Naus [1978] have speculated that the active rehearsal of older children and adults is effective in mediating recall because the intermixing of stimuli during input creates multiple associations among the to-be-remembered items. To the extent that this stimulus intermixing leads to the establishment of an organizational structure, it would be predicted that the effects of active rehearsal would be minimized when subjects are presented with highly structured material to remember. For example, given a stimulus list with a strong built-in organization (such as taxonomic categories presented in blocked order), subjects who are aware of these relationships should be able to use this provided organization to structure their memorization attempts, thus minimizing the advantage of an active rehearsal strategy. In our own research, two experiments examine the role of rehearsal as the stimulus materials differ in the obviousness of the experimenter-provided organization.

In the first of these experiments [*Ornstein* et al., 1975; experiment II], third, sixth, and ninth graders were required to rehearse aloud while memorizing a set of taxonomically related materials. Half of the children received the words in random order, whereas the remaining subjects were presented the items in blocked fashion. Under both conditions, recall increased with age, primarily in the initial and middle serial positions of the lists. Paralleling these differences in recall were corresponding changes in rehearsal activity, seemingly replicating the findings of *Ornstein* et al. [1975; experiment I] with unrelated materials. However, close inspection of the recall and rehearsal patterns showed that the third graders rehearsed in a passive, single-item fashion under both random and blocked presentation conditions, but that this recall was superior under conditions of blocked presentation. These data suggested that a strong preexperimental organization can effect recall directly, without being mediated by means of an active rehearsal strategy.

A conceptual replication of this knowledge base effect was provided by *Ornstein* et al. [1977a] who presented sixth graders with stimulus materials which varied in the salience of list organization. Subjects were instructed to rehearse aloud either using a passive (one-item) rehearsal strategy or an active (multiple-item) rehearsal strategy. The stimulus materials were either unrelated words, related words randomly presented, or related words presented in a blocked fashion. The data were basically consistent with those of *Ornstein* et al. [1975]. The finding that third graders rehearsing passively showed increased recall under conditions of salient list organization was replicated with sixth graders instructed to rehearse passively, in that their recall of blocked items was superior to the recall of the less saliently organized materials. In addition, extending the generality of the previous findings, similar effects were observed with sixth graders instructed to rehearse actively. These data emphasize the limitations of studying mnemonic processes in isolation from knowledge base information and indicate boundary conditions concerning the efficacy of various rehearsal strategies. However, as *Ornstein and Naus* [in press] point out, we have little information concerning how these knowledge base effects are mediated.

Additional work in our laboratory explores the conditions under which the level of rehearsal activity may be influenced by the current contents of the knowledge base, as reflected in the organizational structure of the to-be-remembered materials. For example, *Stone* et al. [1977] instructed second and sixth graders to rehearse aloud as they sorted items into groups defined according to taxonomic, thematic, or randomly generated categories. In addition, for half of the subjects, the contents of each sorting group were visible after placement of each item, whereas for the remaining subjects this was not the case, and only the most recently sorted item in each group was visible. Under both of these presentation conditions, the general pattern of the data is that when subjects were sorting into meaningful groups – both taxonomic or thematic – their rehearsal was more active than when the items were grouped into randomly defined categories. As would be expected, the recall data directly paralleled changes in rehearsal activity. These data suggest that some presentation conditions allow information available in the knowledge base to lead to use of a more efficient strategy which in turn leads to greater recall.

As we have previously suggested [*Ornstein and Naus*, in press], the growing knowledge base may contribute to the increasingly more sophisticated rehearsal strategies employed by older children. In most of our previous work, our focus has been on the spontaneous rehearsal children employ when studying lists of stimulus items that are well-known to subjects of all ages. However, it seems quite possible that the older children may have a more sophisticated understanding of the to-be-remembered items we have studied. If the stimulus materials are more 'meaningful' (in terms of associations and nuance) for the older children than for the younger subjects, this could account at least in part for their tendency to use more active rehearsal strategies. This notion of stimulus knowledge contributing to the use of active rehearsal strategies could be examined directly in de-

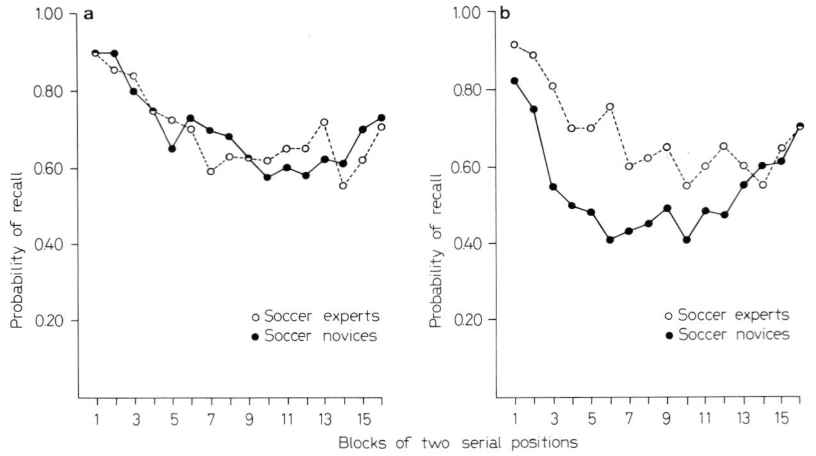

Fig. 4. Mean proportion of taxonomic materials (*a*) and soccer-related materials (*b*) recalled, as a function of serial position for adult soccer experts and novices [from *Naus and Ornstein*, in preparation].

velopmental work in which the characteristics of the stimulus materials are directly manipulated. Alternatively, this issue can be studied indirectly by comparing adult experts and novices in a specific knowledge domain in a memory task involving recall of information from this domain.

Because our developmental studies are still in progress, we will report here the results of an experiment examining the rehearsal and recall of adult experts and novices in the game of soccer. *Naus and Ornstein* [in preparation] presented college students with two different types of categorized work lists to rehearse and recall. One set of materials was composed of words from typical taxonomic categories such as animals, vehicles, and foods, whereas the other set was drawn from the lexicon of the game of soccer, with categories such as types of moves, plays, and kicks. The subjects differed in their knowledge of the soccer-related materials and were selected on the basis of scores on a paper-and-pencil test dealing with soccer, as well as degree of soccer playing experience. Given this novice/expert classification, the soccer materials permitted a knowledge base manipulation in that, although the words were known to all of the subjects, the two groups differed in terms of the meaningfulness of the items and the salience of the categorical structure. The taxonomic materials served as a

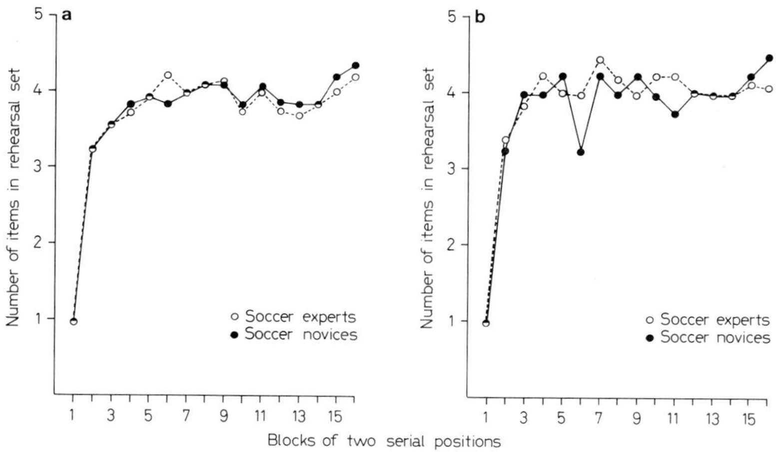

Fig. 5. Mean number of different taxonomic (*a*) and soccer-related (*b*) items per rehearsal set, as a function of serial position for adult soccer experts and novices [from *Naus and Ornstein*, in preparation].

control condition in that both soccer experts and novices were equally familiar with these items. With both types of list, the subjects were informed that the to-be-remembered items could be grouped, but that the words would be presented randomly.

The basic recall data, recall probability as a function of serial position are presented in figure 4. As expected, it is clear in figure 4a that there were no differences between soccer experts and novices in the recall of the taxonomic materials. In contrast, in figure 4b we see that these groups differed markedly in their recall of the soccer-related materials, with recall superiority being observed for the soccer experts, particularly in the initial and middle serial positions. The corresponding rehearsal activity data are presented in figure 5. Again, as expected, we see that there were no differences in the number of different items included in each rehearsal set by the two groups of subjects when learning the taxonomic items. Comparable data are shown in figure 5b in that, somewhat surprisingly, the soccer experts and novices did not differ according to this measure of rehearsal activity when presented with the soccer-related materials.

Probing for more subtle effects of knowledge upon memory strategies, *Naus and Ornstein* [in preparation] examined the extent to which subjects were able to utilize the organizational structure of the lists in their

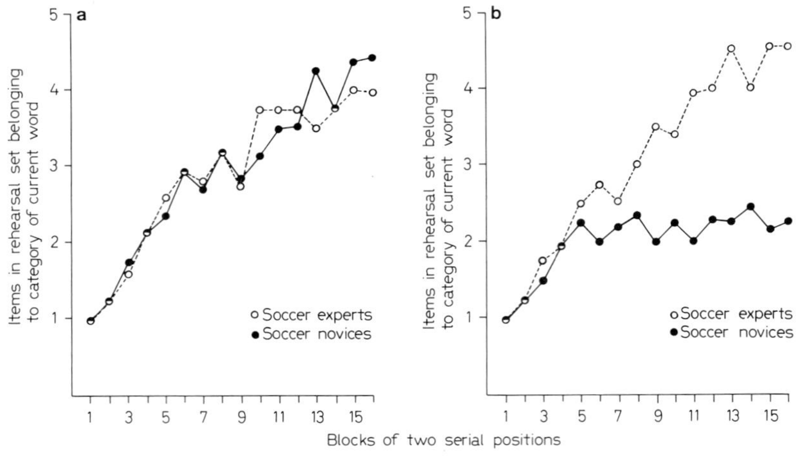

Fig. 6. Mean number of different taxonomic (*a*) and soccer-related (*b*) items per rehearsal set belonging to the category of the currently presented word, as a function of serial position for adult soccer experts and novices [from *Naus and Ornstein*, in preparation].

rehearsal. These data are shown in figure 6. Here are plotted the numbers of items belonging to the category of the currently presented items that are included in the subjects' rehearsal sets. In figure 6a we see that the experts and novices did not differ with the taxonomic materials in terms of the degree to which items from the category of the presented word were included in their rehearsal groupings. Both groups of subjects were able to include previously presented category exemplars to a considerable extent. In contrast, figure 6b demonstrates substantial differences between the groups in terms of the rehearsal of soccer-related materials. The performance of the experts with these lists was very similar to that with the taxonomic materials, whereas the novices were not as able to include in their rehearsal groupings related items that had been presented earlier. The curve for the experts continues to rise with increasing serial position but, in contrast, that for the novices levels off at about two items.

These data suggest that extended familiarity with to-be-remembered materials, perhaps resulting in stronger inter-item associations, may be critical for the maximally efficient execution of active rehearsal techniques. Although this experiment provides the first demonstration of differences in knowledge of stimulus items leading to variations in the form of rehearsal employed, it must be noted that even such a major variation in knowledge as this has rather subtle effects upon rehearsal. Indeed, the differences observed were not in the level of activity observed, but rather in the use of organization in active rehearsal. Further, it must be pointed out that as in previous studies, expertise is simply documented, rather than experimentally created or even qualitatively described in some detail. Finally, although this study has implications for the development of memory, these inferences need to be supported by a series of developmental investigations.

Organizational Strategies

Comparable effects of the knowledge base upon mnemonic strategies can be demonstrated through an investigation of active organizational techniques. For example, *Corsale and Ornstein* [1980] presented third and seventh graders several sorting trials with relatively unrelated materials, prior to a recall test. Seventh graders sorted identically regardless of whether they were asked to form groups that would help them to remember the words or to sort on the basis of meaning. In contrast, third graders asked to group in preparation for recall sorted in a seemingly random fashion, whereas those instructed to group on the basis of meaning sorted in an organizational fashion similar to the seventh graders. Recall performance was always a function of the degree of organization represented in the sorting pattern, regardless of the intent to remember. Thus, as discussed above in the treatment of the organizational literature, third graders instructed to form meaningful groups remembered more than those asked to sort in preparation for recall.

Corsale and Ornstein's [1980] data suggest that third graders have difficulties in responding in a strategic fashion under instructions to remember, but do have the semantic information in permanent memory to group items in a highly organized way. Further, as was seen with children's rehearsal strategies, there may be a gradation in the use of sophisticated mnemonic techniques. Under certain conditions, such as with highly salient stimulus materials, even young children might use active organizational strategies. Confirmation of this viewpoint is seen in *Corsale's* [1978] demonstration that when presented with taxonomically related items in a sort/recall task, third graders sorted spontaneously in a categorically based fashion even under instructions to remember. The contrasting findings of the two experiments of *Corsale* [1978] and *Corsale and Ornstein* [1980] suggest the implementation of a deliberate organizational strategy is not content free, but rather depends upon the nature of the to-be-remembered materials to which the strategy is applied.

Thus far, demonstrations of the effects of the knowledge base on mnemonic strategy utilization have been seen in the cases of rehearsal strategies and organizational (sorting) strategies in preparation for recall. In both of these situations, the mnemonic techniques have been invoked by subjects during study periods prior to attempts at recall. Similar demonstrations of knowledge base effects can be seen with regard to category clustering in recall, but these can also raise serious questions about the fundamental definition of subject-controlled strategies. (See discussion above concerning the problems of identifying mnemonic strategies.) An example of this line of investigation is seen in *Bjorklund and Zeman's* [1982] contrast of first, third, and fifth graders' performance in tasks testing the memory of the names of classmates in addition to taxonomic items. Typical developmental trends in both recall and clustering were observed with the taxonomic materials, whereas minimal differences across age were seen in tests of classmate recall, and performance with these materials was uniformly high. Thus, when asked to remember the names of highly salient and meaningful stimuli (i.e. friends in class), even young children were able to use a clustering at recall strategy.

In discussing this important finding, *Bjorklund and Zeman* [1982] raised the issue of whether the clustering they observed represents a deliberately utilized strategy, or whether the children were generating items in meaningful groups according to some automatic type of process. That the latter might indeed be the case is suggested by their metamemory questionnaire data which indicated very low levels of subject awareness concerning the groups and categories that were actually present in the children's recall protocols. *Bjorklund and Zeman* [1982], in fact, relate their results to *Lange's* [1973, 1978] hypothesis, discussed above, concerning the automatic nature of category clustering as a function of strong preexperimental associations, in preadolescent children. The work of *Bjorklund and Zeman* [1982] and *Lange* [1973, 1978] suggests that in some situations what would appear to be the operation of deliberate strategies may in fact reflect the more-or-less automatic influence of the knowledge base.

The Knowledge Base: an Overview

The *Bjorklund and Zeman* [1982] and *Ornstein* et al. [1975; experiment II] studies report two different knowledge base effects, both of which contrast with the bulk of the demonstrations discussed above. In both of these studies there seem to be automatic effects of the subjects' knowledge, but these effects are somewhat different. In the *Ornstein* et al. [1975]

experiment we see the influence of the knowledge base without any observable strategy component, whereas in the *Bjorklund and Zeman* [1982] study we see what would appear to be a memory strategy but which in all probably is not one. In contrast, in the other experiments discussed here, particularly the *Stone* et al. [1977] rehearsal and sorting study, the *Naus and Ornstein* [in preparation] experiment with soccer-related materials, and the *Corsale* [1978] and *Corsale and Ornstein* [1980] experiments, we have seen memory strategy usage being affected by knowledge base variables. The contrast among these different examples of knowledge base influence raises some fundamental issues concerning the dynamics of the changing knowledge base and its effects on memory performance. As *Ornstein and Naus* [in press] point out, there would appear to be both direct (i.e. non-mediated) effects of the knowledge base and those that are indirect (i.e. strategy mediated).

Perhaps it would be useful to consider a continuum of memory-related activities, ranging from simple mnemonic techniques such as labeling on the one hand, to high-level automatic processes such as the formation of inferences on the other. Given such a conceptualization, it is clear that the influence of the knowledge base upon memory performance cannot be specified in a simple fashion. Rather, it seems likely that the effects of stored knowledge will vary, depending upon the nature of the memory processes involved in the task at hand. For example, it may be quite appropriate to study the development of labeling strategies in young children in isolation of knowledge base effects because these techniques may be robust and not subject to variations as a function of the to-be-remembered stimuli. In contrast, when more sophisticated aspects of verbal rehearsal are investigated (as, for example, the use of organization in rehearsal), it may be difficult to characterize the strategy without taking into consideration the nature of the subject's knowledge of the materials. Finally, when dealing with highly over-practiced and seemingly automatic processes such as categorization and inferencing [*Naus and Halasz,* 1979], it may be impossible to find external indicators of knowledge-base effects, given that these effects may not be mediated at all by deliberate memory strategies.

It is also interesting to speculate that the knowledge base affects memory performance in another way, by influencing the actual emergence of skilled memory strategies. As suggested by *Bjorklund and Zeman* [1982], the implementation of skilled memorizing may follow from experiencing the successful memorial consequences of the automatic or accidental use of a strategy. Thus, for example, the use of clustering as a deliberate strategy may develop as a consequence of previous experiences with automatic clustering and enhanced recall that result from high interstimulus associations. The more general implication of this argument is that developmental changes in the knowledge base, and the direct effects upon memory performance of this articulation, may actually serve as precursors of the skilled use of deliberate mnemonic strategies. Of course, the distinction between deliberate and automatic processes remains a difficult one, and the relationship between these classes may depend upon the level of analysis selected. Thus, certain automatic processes, as hypothesized, may bring about the subsequent appearance of deliberate techniques, but, in addition, extended practice with deliberate procedures may result in their automatization [*Naus and Halasz,* 1979; *Schneider and Shiffrin,* 1977; *Shiffrin and Schneider,* 1977].

It is obvious that much additional systematic work investigating the interrelationships between memory processes and the knowledge base is required. To begin to understand the operation of the knowledge base it is necessary to examine its effects upon memory performance across the broad continuum described above. Thus, the influence of the changing knowledge base upon both simple and complex mnemonic strategies, as well as more automatic memory processes, must be studied. Further, longitudinal work needs to be initiated so that the presumed automatic precursors of deliberate memory strategies can be explored. In addition, the knowledge base cannot be characterized as a dichotic contrast between experts and novices; instead, the interrelationships among its various changing components have to be specified in some detail. Finally, procedures must be developed in which subjects of different ages are systematically exposed to new bodies of knowledge, so that the typical confounding between age and degree of knowledge is eliminated.

Postscript

In our view, the substantial body of data concerning the development of memory strategies that was gathered in the decade since the *Flavell* [1971] symposium now makes it possible to address the four major unanswered questions outlined in this paper. It should be apparent that these issues are interrelated in that they deal with different aspects of the broad question of how the child comes to be skilled at using what he or she knows to process and remember incoming information in an effective fashion. A search for the factors affecting the emergence of skilled memorizing techniques leads directly to longitudinal research in a variety of mnemonic contexts. Further, an adequate characterization of the precursors of skilled strategy usage involves attention to the varied influences of the changing knowledge system on both automatic and deliberate memory processes. Our understanding of the child's growing competence as an efficient processor of information requires attention to these critical issues.

References

Atkinson, R.C.; Shiffrin, R.M.: Human memory: a proposed system and its control processes; in Spence, Spence, The psychology of learning and motivation, vol. 2, pp. 328–372 (Academic Press, New York 1968).

Atkinson, R.C.; Shiffrin, R.M.: The control of short-term memory. Sci. Am. *228:* 82–90 (1971).

Baker-Ward, L.: Young children's intentional memory behavior in a recall task. Proc. Southeastern Conf. on Human Development, Alexandria 1980.

Belmont, J.M.; Butterfield, E.C.: What the development of short-term memory is. Hum. Dev. *14:* 236–248 (1971).

Best, D.L.: Inducing children to generate mnemonic organizational strategies in recall; unpublished doct. diss., Chapel Hill (1981).

Best, D.L.; Ornstein, P.A.: Children's generation and communication of organizational strategies. Proc. of the Society for Research in Child Development, San Francisco 1979.

Bjorklund, D.F.; Ornstein, P.A.; Haig, J.R.: Developmental differences in organization and recall: training in the use of organizational techniques. Devl Psychol. *13:* 175–183 (1977).

Bjorklund, D.F.; Zeman, B.R.: Children's organization and metamemory awareness in their recall of familiar information. Child Dev. *53:* 799–810 (1982).

Bransford, J.D.; Nitsch, K.E.; Franks, J.J.: Schooling and the facilitation of knowing; in Anderson, Spiro, Montague, Schooling and the acquisition of knowledge, pp. 31–55 (Erlbaum, Hillsdale 1977).

Brown, A.L.: The development of memory: knowing, knowing about knowing, knowing how to know; in Reese, Advances in child development and behavior, vol. 10, pp. 104–152 (Academic Press, New York 1975).

Brown, A.L.: Theories of memory and the problems of development: activity, growth, and knowledge; in Craik, Cermak, Levels of processing and memory (Erlbaum, Hillsdale 1979).

Chase, W.G.; Simon, H.A.: The mind's eye in chess; in Chase, Visual information processing, pp. 215–281 (Academic Press, New York 1973).

Chi, M.T.H.: Age differences in memory span. J. exp. Child Psychol. *23:* 266–281 (1977).

Chi, M.T.H.: Knowledge structure and memory development; in Siegler, Children's thinking: What develops? pp. 73–96 (Erlbaum, Hillsdale 1978).

Cole, M.; Scribner, S.: Culture and thought (Wiley, New York 1974).

Corsale, K.: Factors affecting children's use of organization in recall; unpublished doct. diss., Chapel Hill (1978).
Corsale, K.; Ornstein, P.A.: Developmental changes in children's use of semantic information in recall. J. exp. Child Psychol. *30:* 231–245 (1980).
Corsini, D.A.: Memory: Interaction of stimulus and organismic factors. Hum. Dev. *14:* 227–235 (1971).
Craik, F.I.M.; Lockhart, R.S.: Levels of processing: a framework for memory research. J. verb. Learn. verb. Behav. *11:* 671–684 (1972).
Feurstein, R.: Instrumental enrichment (University Park Press, Baltimore 1980).
Flavell, J.H.: Developmental studies of mediated memory; in Reese, Lipsitt, Advances in child development and behavior, vol. 5, pp. 182–211 (Academic Press, New York 1970).
Flavell, J.H.: What is memory development the development of? Hum. Dev. *14:* 225–286 (1971).
Flavell, J.H.; Wellman, H.M.: Metamemory; in Kail, Hagen, Perspectives on the development of memory and cognition, pp. 3–33 (Erlbaum, Hillsdale 1977).
Hagen, J.W.: Some thoughts on how children learn to remember. Hum. Dev. *14:* 262–271 (1971).
Haith, H.M.: Developmental changes in visual information processing and short-term visual memory. Hum. Dev. *14:* 249–261 (1971).
Hasher, L.; Zacks, R.T.: Automatic and effortful processes in memory. J. exp. Psychol. *108:* 356–388 (1979).
Hyde, T.S.; Jenkins, J.J.: The differential effects of incidental tasks on the organization of recall of a list of highly associated words. J. exp. Psychol. *82:* 472–481 (1969).
Istomina, Z.M.: The development of voluntary memory in preschool-age children. Soviet Psychol. *13:* 5–64 (1975).
Johnson, S.C.: Hierarchical clustering schemes. Psychometrika *32:* 241–254 (1967).
Kail, R.V.: The development of memory in children (Freeman, San Francisco 1979).
Kreutzer, M.A.; Leonard, C.; Flavell, J.H.: An interview study of children's knowledge about memory. Monogr. Soc. Res. Child Dev. *40* (1975).
Lange, G.: The development of conceptual and rote recall skills among school-age children. J. exp. Child Psychol. *15:* 394–407 (1973).
Lange, G.: Organization-related processes in children's recall; in Ornstein, Memory development in children, pp. 101–128 (Erlbaum, Hillsdale 1978).
Levin, J.R.; Yussen, S.R.; De Rose, T.M.; Pressley, M.: Developmental changes in assessing recall and recognition memory capacity. Devl Psychol. *13:* 608–615 (1977).
Liberty, C.; Ornstein, P.A.: Age differences in organization and recall: the effects of training in categorization. J. exp. Child Psychol. *15:* 169–186 (1973).
Lindberg, M.A.: Is knowledge-base development a necessary and sufficient condition for memory development? J. exp. Child Psychol. *30:* 401–410 (1980).
Luria, A.R.: Cognitive development: its cultural and social foundations (Harvard University Press, Cambridge 1976).
Mandler, G.: Organization and memory; in Spence, Spence, The psychology of learning and motivation, vol. 1, pp. 328–372 (Academic Press, New York 1967).
Medlin, R.: Memory in the elementary school; unpublished manuscript, Chapel Hill (1978).
Miller, S.A.; Brownwell, C.A.; Zukier, H.: Cognitive certainty in children: effects of con-

cept, developmental level, and method of assessment. Devl Psychol. *13:* 236–245 (1977).

Myers, N.A.; Perlmutter, M.: Memory in the years from two to five; in Ornstein, Memory development in children, pp. 191–218 (Erlbaum, Hillsdale 1978).

Naus, M.J.; Halasz, F.: Developmental perspectives on cognitive processing and semantic memory structure; in Craik, Cermak, Levels of processing and memory, pp. 258–288 (Erlbaum, Hillsdale 1979).

Naus, M.J.; Ornstein, P.A.: Rehearsal and recall of categorical materials by experts and novices (in preparation).

Naus, M.J.; Ornstein, P.A.; Aivano, S.: Developmental changes in memory: the effects of processing time and rehearsal instruction. J. exp. Child Psychol. *23:* 237–251 (1977a).

Naus, M.J.; Ornstein, P.A.; Hoving, K.L.: Developmental implications of multi-store and depth of processing models of memory; in Ornstein, Memory development in children, pp. 219–231 (Erlbaum, Hillsdale 1978).

Naus, M.J.; Ornstein, P.A.; Kreshtool, K.: Developmental differences in recall and recognition: the relationship between rehearsal and memory as test expectations changes. J. exp. Child Psychol. *23:* 252–265 (1977b).

Ornstein, P.A.; Corsale, K.: Organizational factors in children's memory; in Puff, Memory organization and structure, pp. 219–257 (Academic Press, New York 1979a).

Ornstein, P.A.; Corsale, K.: Process and structure in children's memory; in Whitehurst, Zimmerman, The functions of language and cognition, pp. 199–228 (Academic Press, New York 1979b).

Ornstein, P.A.; Naus, M.J.: Rehearsal processes in children's memory; in Ornstein, Memory development in children, pp. 69–99 (Erlbaum, Hillsdale 1978).

Ornstein, P.A.; Naus, M.J.: Effects of the knowledge base on children's memory processing; in Sidowski, Conditioning, cognition, and methodology: contemporary issues in experimental psychology (Erlbaum, Hillsdale, in press).

Ornstein, P.A.; Naus, M.J.; Liberty, C.: Rehearsal and organizational processes in children's memory. Child Dev. *46:* 818–830 (1975).

Ornstein, P.A.; Naus, M.J.; Miller, T.D.: The effects of list organization and rehearsal activity in memory. Child Dev. *48:* 292–295 (1977a).

Ornstein, P.A.; Naus, M.J.; Stone, B.P.: Rehearsal training and developmental differences in memory. Devl Psychol. *13:* 15–24 (1977b).

Paris, S.G.: Coordination of means and goals in the development of mnemonic skills; in Ornstein, Memory development in children, pp. 259–273 (Erlbaum, Hillsdale 1978a).

Paris, S.G.: The development of inference and transformation as memory operations; in Ornstein, Memory development in children, pp. 129–156 (Erlbaum, Hillsdale 1978b).

Perlmutter, M.: Children's memory; in Perlmutter, New directions for child development (Jossey-Bass, San Francisco 1980).

Peterson, C.R.: Age changes in the effects of processing tasks on pictorial recognition memory; unpublished doct. diss., Chapel Hill (1977).

Piaget, J.; Inhelder, B.: Memory and intelligence (Basic Books, New York 1973).

Ratner, H.H.; Myers, N.A.: Related picture cues and memory for hidden-object locations at age two. Child Dev. *51:* 561–564 (1980).

Richman, C.L.; Nida, S.; Pittman, L.: Effects of meaningfulness on child free-recall learning. Devl Psychol. *12:* 460–465 (1976).

Rundus, D.: Analysis of rehearsal processes in free recall. J. exp. Psychol. *89:* 63–77 (1971).
Rundus, D.; Atkinson, R.C.: Rehearsal processes in free recall: a procedure for direct observation. J. verb. Learn. verb. Behav. *9:* 97–105 (1970).
Schneider, W.; Shiffrin, R.M.: Controlled and automatic human information processing. I. Detection, search, and attention. Psychol. Rev. *84:* 1–66 (1977).
Sharp, D.; Cole, M.; Lave, C.: Education and cognitive development: the evidence from experimental research. Monogr. Soc. Res. Child Dev. *44* (1979).
Shiffrin, R.M.; Schneider, W.: Controlled and automatic human information processing. II. Perceptual learning, automatic attending, and a general theory. Psychol. Rev. *84:* 127–190 (1977).
Smirnov, A.A.: Problems of the psychology of memory (Plenum Publishing, New York 1973).
Stern, J.W.; Neubauer, A.L.; Dennig, L.; Ornstein, P.A.; Naus, M.J.: The effects of task performance on the prediction and assessment of children's memory abilities: the interaction of metamemory and memory behavior (in preparation).
Stone, B.P.; Naus, M.J.; Ornstein, P.A.: An analysis of active rehearsal in children's memory. Proc. Meet. of the American Psychological Association, San Francisco 1977.
Wagner, D.A.: Memories of Morocco: the influence of age, schooling, and environment on memory. Cognitive Psychol. *10:* 1028 (1978).
Weiss, S.L.; Robinson, G.; Hastie, R.: The relationship of depth of processing to free recall in second and fourth graders. Devl Psychol. *13:* 525–526 (1977).
Wellman, H.M.: The early development of intentional memory behavior. Hum. Dev. *20:* 86–101 (1977).
Wellman, H.M.; Johnson, C.N.: Understanding of mental processes: a developmental study of 'remember' and 'forget'. Child Dev. *50:* 79–88 (1979).
Yussen, S.R.; Levy, V.M.: Developmental changes in predicting one's own span of short-term memory. J. exp. Child Psychol. *19:* 502–508 (1975).
Yussen, S.R.; Paquette, N.S.: Developmental changes in predicting recognition memory for semantically related and unrelated sentences. Devl Psychol. *14:* 107–113 (1978).

Contr. hum. Dev., vol. 9, pp. 31–51 (Karger, Basel 1983)

Metamemory Revisited

Henry M. Wellman[1]
University of Michigan, Ann Arbor, Mich., USA

It was a decade ago, at this symposium's predecessor, that metamemory made its conceptual entry into our midst [*Flavell*, 1971]. Since that time, and especially in the last 5 years, metamemory and its broader namesake metacognition have become established constructs in developmental psychology. Developmental journals and meetings are replete with investigation, discussion, or, at least, mention of metacognition. The present tenth-year review seems an opportune time to consider the current 'substance' of metamemory, as well as its prospects.

A comprehensive review of metamemory would consider in depth at least four questions: (a) How should metamemory be defined or conceptualized? (b) What is our best developmental description of the acquisition of metamnemonic knowledge? (c) What mechanisms or larger processes and developments account for and influence the development of metamemory? (d) What role does metamemory play in memory development and in various memory performances? I cannot address all of these questions. I will touch on only two: What is metamemory and what is its role?

Perhaps it goes without saying, but a symposium like this provides an author with a much needed but all too rare opportunity for egocentrism and self-indulgence. Thus, you should be forewarned that these remarks are not intended as an exhaustive analysis of metamemory, but represent my current opinion and hunches about what metamemory development is, and is not, the development of. In addition, while my primary goal is to discuss metamemory, in some cases it will be impossible or needlessly inefficient to extricate metamemory narrowly from metacognition more

[1] Preparation of this paper was supported in part by NIMH Grant MH 35058 to the author.

broadly. Indeed I hope that my remarks, even when focused on metamemory, will have application to the larger domain.

What Is Metamemory?

Let me begin by considering what is metamemory, or more broadly metacognition? There are two different answers to this question: First, from the point of view of the investigator studying memory, metamemory is not a precise psychological construct; it is a fuzzy concept. Second, from the point of view of the child acquiring metamemory, metamemory is not a collection of facts about memory, but an intricately interwoven system of knowledge.

Metamemory from the Researcher's Point of View

Consider first: What is metamemory from the researcher's point of view? The standard definition of metamemory comes in two parts. There is the statement that metamemory is the person's knowledge about memory. Next, this statement is accompanied by citing various obvious instances of metamemory, examples of knowledge about memory tasks, about memory strategies, about personal memory abilities and states. There has been recent dissatisfaction with this definition by extension, and calls for a more precise intensional definition [*Cavanaugh and Perlmutter*, 1982; *Paris*, 1978]. What is requested here is specification of the distinctive attributes which clearly distinguish the 'metas' from the not, and which will define what all metamemories have in common. Underlying the need for definition is a frustration: How can metamemory be studied, measured, and especially evaluated if we do not know exactly what it is? Notice that this frustration, and the desire for precise definition, rest on the implicit assumption that whatever metamemory is, it can be considered a well-defined category. On the contrary my view is that metamemory, or metacognition, is an ill-defined category, a fuzzy concept.

By identifying metacognition as a fuzzy concept I wish to emphasize four features of its definition. First, the concept encompasses an essential, central distinction. However, this distinction serves to anchor the concept, not intensionally define it. Second, prototypic central instances of the concept are easily recognized. However, third, at the periphery, agreement as to whether an activity is legitimately metacognition breaks down; the definitional boundaries are truly fuzzy. Related to this, and fourth, different processes all of which partake of the original distinction may be related only loosely one to another. Thus, the term metacognition or metamemory serves primarily to designate a complex of associated phenomena.

The central distinction involved is, of course, the distinction between remembering versus having knowledge about memory. That is, generally, the difference is between engaging in some form of cognition versus knowledge of that cognition itself. This distinction is a fundamental and a classic one. Philosophers and psychologists have long been interested in human consciousness and reflection, terms which are based in part on the same essential distinction. This distinction is also a straightforward one in the sense that prototypic instances of knowledge about cognition, as distinct from engaging in the activity itself, are easy to generate or conceive. Obvious examples include tip of the tongue knowledge – where someone knows about his or her cognition in spite of inability to execute the cognitive act right then – and knowing that rehearsal aids short-term memory, without currently engaging in rehearsal itself. Indeed the ease of access to these prototypic instances probably accounts for why metamemory originally caught on so quickly.

As is typical of ill-defined concepts, however, when we progress away from central instances agreement breaks down and what is and what is not 'meta' becomes obscure. As an example of this consider table I, which presents a biased but informed sample of views about metamemory/metacognition. The four categories of phenomena in the left hand column represent different types of knowledge and awareness about memory or cognition. The first, factual knowledge about memory, includes, for example, knowing that recall is harder than recognition, that organized lists are easier to remember than unorganized ones, that rehearsal improves short-term recall and so on. The second category involves cognitive assessments of one's own current memory, such as feeling-of-knowing judgments ('I know I know that'), assessments of comprehension difficulty ('I didn't get that') and so on. The third category concerns the intelligent employment of cognition. It is knowledge about cognition in the sense of a skill, or knowing how to execute various procedures to cope with cognitive tasks such as remembering. Finally, there are cognitive feelings or affective assessments and reactions to various cognitive performances, such as amazement that you got the right answer, puzzlement about an outcome, elation at a successful cognitive endeavor.

While consideration of different types of metacognition is informative in itself, it is the fact, captured in table I, that the term metacognition is

Table I. Metacognition

	Flavell [1978, 1979]	*Baker and Brown* [in press]	*Wellman* [in press]
1. Factual, long-term knowledge about cognitive tasks, processes, strategies, etc.	metacognitive knowledge[a]	metacognitive knowledge[a]	the person's theory of mind[a]
2. Knowledge of one's own current memory states, contents, limits	metacognitive experiences[a]	metacognitive knowledge[a]	cognitive monitoring[a]
3. Regulation, control of cognitive processes, strategies	cognitive monitoring[a]	metacognitive skills, activities[a]	possible applied use of metacognition (1, 2 above) in various situations, tasks
4. Conscious cognitive feelings (curious, puzzled), affective states related to cognitive activity	metacognitive experiences[a]	?	?

[a] Included as metacognition by the writer.

applied to these classes differently by the different authors which is most pertinent to the present discussion. Notice that consistent with a fuzzy conception there is good agreement as to the metacognitive status of some, presumably central, instances (classes 1 and 2 in table I), but considerable disagreement or uncertainty about other instances. Further, closer examination of the four distinct categories suggests that these various types of metacognition probably do not possess a unique set of critical features. They are all knowledge, under some understanding of that term, and they all refer to or are distinct from the focal cognitive act itself. But they also remain distinctly different sorts of things in many respects. Thus, while the subclasses do relate to the original distinction in various ways, in the end the extended domain probably constitutes an array of different processes linked by family resemblance. Once again this is typical for ill-defined, natural, or fuzzy categories.

Given a concept which cannot be precisely intensionally defined, then definition requires not only discussion of the internal nature of the category but discussion of the concept's place in some larger conceptual space as well. Thus, it is useful to consider, briefly, associated concepts which are related to and allied with the notions of metamemory and metacognition. Obviously, metamemory and such topics as metalanguage, meta-attention, and the metacognitive aspects of reading and mathematics all relate as specific content domains of metacognition in general. At a different level, metacognition itself is one of a family of conceptual bedfellows and partially synonymous constructs. These would include notions such as executive or control processes, planfulness, consciousness or reflection, and recent specific derivatives of these, such as meta-plans [*Wilensky*, 1981] and internal 'critics' or 'specialists' [*Hayes-Roth and Hayes-Roth*, 1979], which inform and regulate other cognitive processes. Further associated constructs are found in social psychology, for example, person perception, self-concepts – especially mental self-concepts – and personal attributions which guide task efforts and persistence. This plethora of overlapping conceptual kin aids in cross-referencing and defining metacognition and, further, indicates the widespread agreement as to the importance of metacognition-like notions and distinctions.

While conceiving of metamemory/metacognition as a fuzzy concept may seem dismayingly imprecise to some, it has its distinct advantages. Most importantly this perspective avoids the futility of striving for precise, intensive definition when in fact what we have is a cover term denoting a host of related processes and knowledge. Further, admitting the imprecision of the general concept still allows, and may even spur, the formation of derivative theoretical constructs of increased precision. Finally, notice that psychology is often in the business of exploring ill-defined categories of processes and effects. As a pertinent example, 10 years ago at this symposium's forerunner, the conclusion was that memory itself was not some one construct, certainly not a unitary mental faculty, but a term applicable to any and all cognitive processes that were recruited or recruitable for the task of storing and retrieving information. Surely that is an ill-defined category if there ever was one. Yet this particular fuzzy conception has fostered, not hindered, our understanding and study of memory development.

The fuzzy-concept perspective on the definition of metamemory has numerous implications. I want to point out just one. In the essential distinction and in the agreed upon prototypic instances, metamemory is fundamentally identified as a form of knowledge. Of course, knowledge is itself a notorious, ill-defined category, but my belief here is that metamemory is indeed essentially knowledge and, further, that this means that it is no different from any other knowledge one possesses [*Flavell*, 1979]. What distinguishes metamemory is its referent – it is knowledge about the human information-processing system. Otherwise it has no special status. It is stored in long term memory like other knowledge; it may be neither more nor less consciously accessible than other knowledge; it has, on the average, no greater nor fewer implications for behavior than other knowledge.

Metamemory from the Knower's Point of View

Identifying metamemory as an instance of the larger construct, knowledge, provides a useful transition to considering the related question: What is metamemory from the point of view of the child or subject? My remarks here are limited to categories 1 and 2 in table I – the categories of metamemory which I take to be the prototypic ones. The main point here is that since these types of metamemory refer to the child's knowledge, then, like all knowledge, the child's metamemory is very likely to be a highly integrated set of notions, propositions, and concepts. Thus, you will see why I have come to use the phrase 'the child's theory of mind' to refer to part of this knowledge [*Wellman*, in press]. The term, theory, unambiguously denotes a set of interrelated propositions and concepts.

Curiously, while there has been considerable concern about how different aspects of metamemory relate *definitionally* for the investigator, there has been little study of how different aspects of metamemory relate *functionally* for the subject – the knower. Most metamemory research has studied either one isolated metamemory fact or judgment and its development, or a set of such discrete facts.

On the assumption that metamemory or metacognition is an integrated theory of mind, my collaborators and I have been trying to investigate this larger naive theory – how various facts and concepts are knit together from the child's viewpoint. We have been tackling this in two distinguishable manners. First, we have been investigating how children integrate information about a number of different memory variables into a larger conception of memory tasks and processes [*Fabricius and Wellman*, 1983; *Wellman*, 1978; *Wellman* et al., 1981]. Second, on the assumption that memory behavior and processes are a subset of all human behaviors, we have studied how the child's understanding of memory and cognition fits into an understanding of human behavior in general [*Johnson and Wellman*, 1982]. The first of these approaches is somewhat bottom-up, starting with conceptions of different memory features and fitting these together; the second approach is more top-down.

Let me elaborate on only the first of these two approaches as an example. A classic question in metamemory research has been: When does the child realize that number – different numbers of items to be remembered – is a memory relevant variable? The typical study involves showing children arrays of increasing or decreasing items and soliciting their judgments as to which they think they could remember perfectly. Many young children seem oblivious to the number presented, saying they will remember all of even the longest list [*Flavell* et al., 1970]. By studying this one variable in isolation, it is possible to conclude that the young child does not know that number influences memory, but that with development this knowledge – metamemory – is acquired.

However the picture is more complex, and interesting, than this. For example, in one study we presented various memory situations to the child and asked how many items would be remembered, but in this case the depicted memory situations varied both in respect to number of items *and* in respect to the effort applied by the memorizer [*Wellman* et al., 1981]. Nine situations were used that represented all possible combinations of three levels of item number (4, 8, and 12 items) crossed with three levels of effort (no, little, and a lot of effort). The children's predictions of how many items would be remembered are in figure 1. It is clear in this data that children integrate information about both number and effort into their metamemory judgments. The lines are separate, indicating that judgments differ by effort *and* the lines all slope downward, indicating that judgments differ by number of items presented.

While children integrate information about both number and effort in their judgments, even more revealing is how they combine these variables together. For example, table II represents the relative weighting of changes in number versus changes in effort in children's judgment. In this ratio the effect of change in effort on performance is in the numerator and the effect of change in number in the denominator. Thus, a large ratio means that effort is seen as more important than number and decreases in the ratio mean decreasing importance of effort coupled with increasing importance of number of items. As table II shows, while effort and number are both understood, effort looms very large in the young child's conception of memory and decreases with age.

This finding of course has implications for the single-variable studies of judgment of number. In the classic task, for example, a young child is

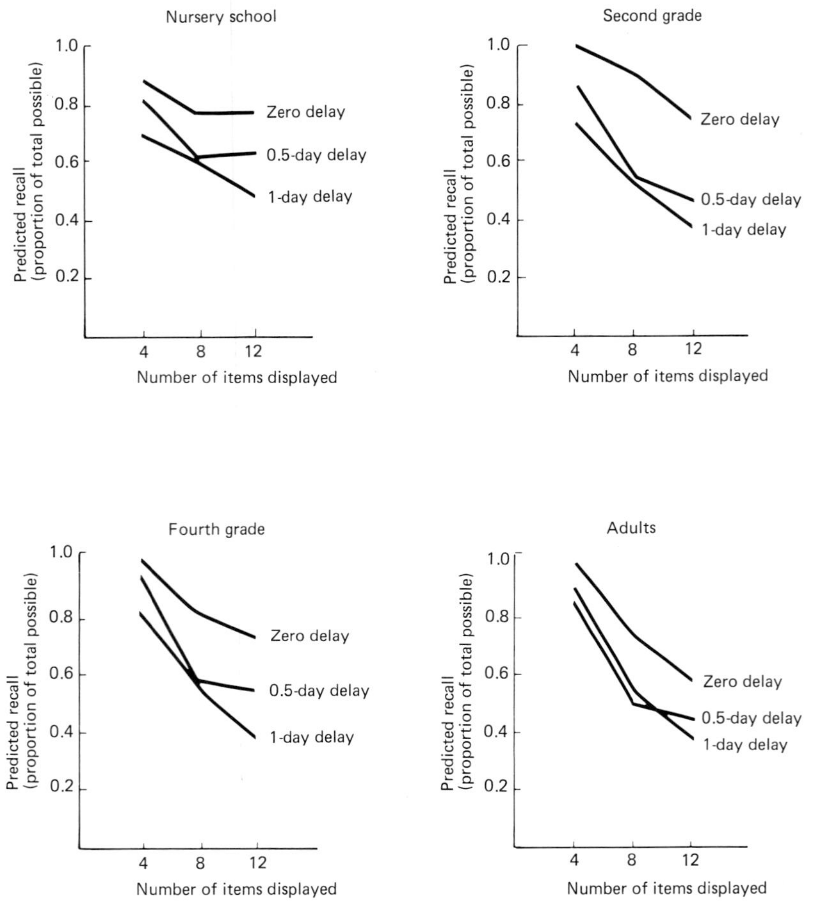

Fig. 1. Predicted recall as a function of items, effort, and age [from *Wellman* et al., 1981].

likely to say he or she could recall longer and longer lists regardless of the number of items simply by implicitly varying effort in his or her judgments: 'Sure I'll remember this list, it's real long but if I just try hard enough I'll get it!'

In short, what a child judges in an isolated metamemory task is only a manifestation of a complex interrelated system of knowledge about memory. Of course, studying all pairwise combinations of all metamemory variables will probably not be much more informative than studying single variables; certainly it will not be any less tedious. Thus, in the larger line of

Table II. Relative importance of number and effort in children's judgments of recall

	Age			
	nursery school	grade 2	grade 4	college
a/b	7.83	6.58	5.36	1.69

a = Change in predicted items recalled with increasing effort. b = Change in predicted items recalled with increasing number of items.

research, what we are trying to do is to study the child's interrelated understanding of (1) number or amount to be remembered, (2) effort or resources expended in remembering, (3) study time or opportunity to study the items and (4) delay from study until test, or retention interval. We have chosen these four particular aspects of memory situations because they are linked to an important larger conception – in this case the larger conception is the child's understanding of memory limits. Number, effort, and time, for example, are the variables that form the basis for contemporary psychological descriptions of memory limitations. Thus, in exploring children's integration of these key factors, we are looking at their conception of memory limitations.

This approach suggests a general strategy for studying children's larger theories of memory. It involves identifying the larger conceptions that lie behind current psychological accounts of memory and studying their development. Much information processing psychology has a heavy intuitive basis – what is the development of similar intuitions in the child? Knowledge and awareness of cognitive limitations is only one such general conception worthy of study.

Metamemory's Role in Memory Performance

Consideration of what metamemory is gives useful background for the second major question: What is metamemory's role, especially its role in ongoing memory performances? Just as there have been increasing calls for precise definition of metamemory, there have been calls for definitive research on whether metamemory is or is not implicated in memory performances. Most of the concern here is about whether metamemory knowledge is instrumental in directing strategic memory behavior. In this regard the present state of affairs looks remarkably similar to analogous concerns about the attitude-behavior relation in social psychology. In that literature there was the early presumption that attitudes must be tightly linked to behavior. This was followed by a growing disenchantment with attitude research altogether, based on demonstrations of low attitude-behavior correlations [*Wicker*, 1969]. At present, the discussion seems to have reached a third phase of renewed interest in attitudes and a reappraisal of the attitude-behavior relation. Attitudes are now proving to be powerful predictors in some but not other situations, as expected on the basis of theoretical considerations [*Ajzen and Fishbein*, 1977; *Cialdini* et al., 1981].

In terms of this three-phase model, current discussion of metamemory seems to be at either the beginning or the height of the disenchantment phase. Based on analogy to attitude-behavior research, this disenchantment seems both inevitable and shortsighted. Some disenchantment seems inevitable because the terms metamemory and metacognition have become rapidly, and often casually, incorporated into a great many explanations of a great many other phenomena. It seems inevitable that when our understanding of metacognition is itself more complete, it will seem not only a fuzzier but also a less powerful, as well as knottier, explanatory concept than some of the explicit and implicit claims made for it. Metamemory will not meet all of our unresolved problems about strategy, consciousness, training and development.

On the other hand, complete disenchantment seems shortsighted. Specifically the growing scepticism about metamemory's role in accounting for memory performance (and its development) should be kept in check. As in the attitude-behavior literature, a cautious, balanced view about when and where specific metamemory knowledge influences corresponding memory activity will probably prevail in the end. In the hopes of advancing this cautious but positive view, I would like to make a few observations about current and future efforts to empirically explore metamemory-memory linkages.

The first thing to say is that many attempts to test metamemory-memory relations are based on what amounts to a straw man, an overly simplistic model of what the relations might be. In essence, the straw model is captured in figure 2. Some piece of meta-knowledge is represented horizontally, and some derivative memory performance or behavior vertically. The idea is that a person either knows this metamnemonic information or

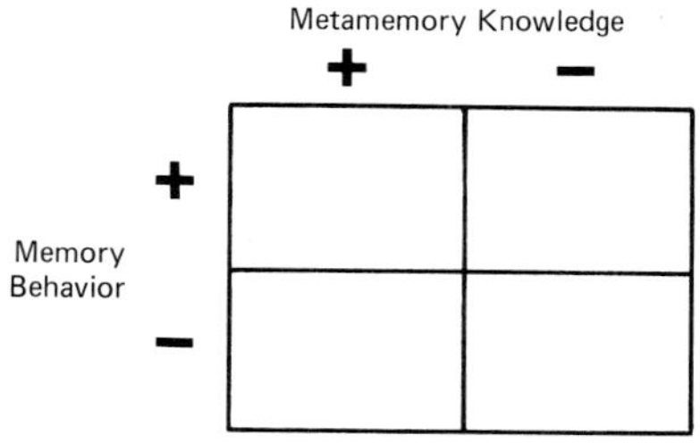

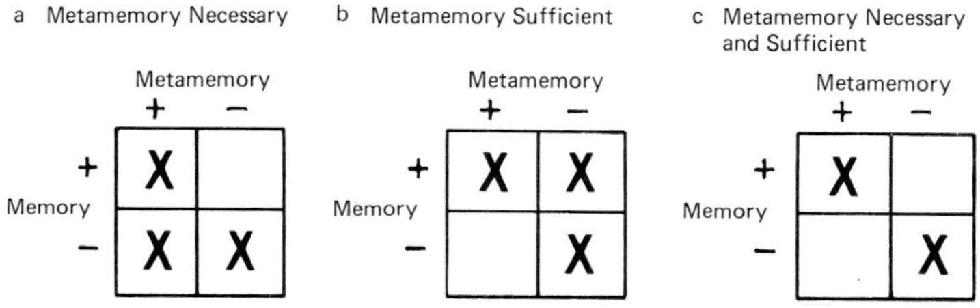

Fig. 2. Possible metamemory-memory relations.

not: for instance, that organized items are easier to recall than unorganized, unrelated items. And the person either performs this sort of behavior or not in suitable memory situations, such as converting an unorganized set of items into an organized set by discovering or creating groups, themes, categories, and so on. If metamemory is influential in memory performance, then there ought to be a correlation between knowledge and action. Indeed, given this model one might even try to determine what specific role metamemory knowledge plays in relation to memory performance. For example, metamemory might be necessary for memory behavior, in which case you would expect a pattern like *a*, or it might be sufficient but not necessary, in which case you get the pattern in *b*, or perhaps both necessary and sufficient in some memory behavior or performance, as in *c*.

I and others have discussed before why this particular analysis yields testable but straw man predictions – why one might never expect to find these relations in real behavior [*Flavell*, 1978; *Flavell and Wellman*, 1977]. For example, a person could know that organization is an effective tactic but think that a particular list is so easy that it only requires quick inspection; a person may recognize that organization is useful if asked about it but be unable to think of it on his or her own; she or he may use organization when being strategic, but the task may fail to evoke strategic activity at all. Rather than to reiterate the problems mentioned in other places, let me advance two new and, I believe, compelling considerations here.

The first consideration brings us back to my earlier remarks. The metamemory knowledge tapped in investigations like this is usually a single metamemory fact (or a list of such facts). Does organization (in some one instantiation) help? Again, this approach ignores the child's larger theory and integrated knowledge of memory, of which it is one slice. For example, suppose the subject says, 'Yes, organization can make memory easier', but then does not employ organization in memory tasks. This, in fact, is the modal negative finding. Recall from the earlier discussion that children know that many factors influence memory but, within a larger conception of memory, may believe that the single most powerful factor is effort. A child with such a theory could both know that organization is better than nothing, in the metamemory assessment, and yet, when faced with the memory task itself, just decide that trying harder is the best strategy. In doing this, the child's memory behavior would indeed be influenced by his or her metamemory, if by that we mean the larger theory of memory. Yet, by correlating knowledge of organization with organizational behavior alone, the opposite conclusion would seem warranted. In short, unsuccessful attempts to correlate single facts and single behaviors seem neither surprising nor compelling. More revealing tests of metamemory's role in memory behavior await an understanding of the integrated system of knowledge about memory which children develop. This is just that type of larger theory of memory of which we have, as yet, little developmental information.

The second set of considerations has to do with the expectation that it is plausible to generate clear data about whether metamemory is necessary and/or sufficient for some memory behavior. [I am indebted to *Cook and Campbell*, 1979, for the following way of presenting this problem.] Suppose that the true state of affairs is something like that in figure 3. In that figure, the general problem is represented by a specific example concerning organization's role in memory performance. There is a continuum of awareness or knowledge about organization's role in memory, which is in fact linked in a very straightforward manner with an increasing likelihood of engaging in various organizational behaviors in storing and retrieving items. Thus, the true relation between knowledge and act is a very tight one. However, any one memory task can present a certain threshold – it

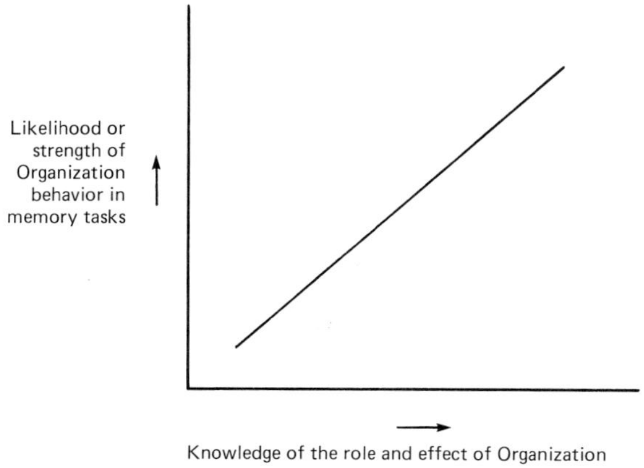

Fig. 3. Ideal metamemory-memory relationship.

will make obvious, say, the presence of organizational behavior, but only at some level or strength. Below that level, persons will not seem to be organizing, above it they will, as indexed on this task. The same is true of metamemory tasks. Different tasks may require more or less knowledge of organization before that knowledge is revealed in the metamemory task itself.

In short, assuming even this artificially tight true relation between behavior and metamemory, one could find evidence for all possibilities just depending on task characteristics. In figure 4, for instance, are shown the three contrasting possibilities talked of before, all observable from the same underlying relationship. Depending on how the tasks capture knowledge and behavior, then, one could find evidence of a necessary but not sufficient relation, a sufficient but not necessary relation or a necessary and sufficient relation. And, of course, if the same tasks are differentially difficult for different individuals, then across a group of subjects it is possible to get the remaining fourth pattern where metamemory seems neither necessary nor sufficient for the behavior to occur.

Finally, to move from critique to data, gloom about low correlations between metamemory and memory is premature; one or two salient negative findings [*Cavanaugh and Borkowski*, 1980; *Salatas and Flavell*, 1976] are often mentioned while other relevant research is overlooked. Specifically, there is ample evidence of at least one intriguing cluster of metamemory and memory behavior links. This evidence comes from investiga-

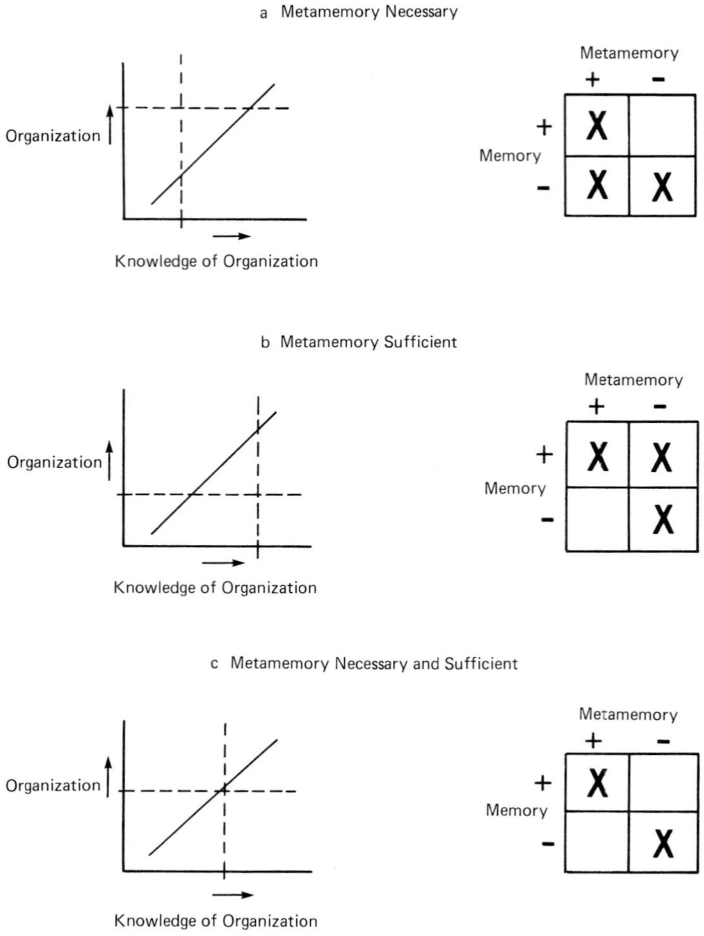

Fig. 4. Possible metamemory-memory relationships derived from different kinds of tasks.

tion of what can be called effort allocation strategies and their development. Much research on memory strategies has concerned specific memory strategies, such as rehearsal, organization, elaboration. However, the memorizer's task can be construed as a general one, requiring the strategic allocation of effort. He or she must do something instead of nothing, do this instead of that, concentrate effort on these items more than those. How might metamemory influence this process? Consider as an example, that in research on feeling-of-knowing judgments [*Wellman*, 1977] even kindergarteners make accurate feeling-of-knowing judgments. If faced with a set of items, none of which they can presently recall, they know which of these are potentially retrievable and which not. That is, they have knowledge of the current state of their own memory, the second type in table I. Is such metamemory knowledge influential in the child's memory behavior? It certainly could be. Optimal retrieval efforts should at some point depend on such knowledge; retrieval effort should be terminated if one can assess in advance that one does not know the items; it can be prolonged if in fact 'you know you know it'. In short, metamemory judgments of this sort could direct one's effort allocation strategies.

With this in mind, a very straightforward demonstration was possible. 24 kindergarteners, 24 first graders and 24 third graders were shown pictures of concrete objects and asked to name them. Those items which were not named were re-presented and the children were asked to judge whether they felt they knew the name anyway, or not. On the basis of these judgments, we can consider all the unnamed items as falling into two groups, those the child thinks he or she knows anyway (feeling-of-knowing + items) and those he or she judges to be not known (feeling-of-knowing − items). After this judgment, the unnamed items were presented to the child again, twice more, for different tasks. In these tasks the child was not asked to name the item, but was asked other questions about the item. During these subsequent presentations, however, the child's behavior was carefully coded for various indications of retrieval effort. The categories of retrieval effort recorded were: *(1) Attempts to name.* Child spontaneously states a potential name or part of a name for the item ('telescope' for binoculars, 'fun... fum...' for funnel). *(2) Retrieves related cue.* Child spontaneously voices a potential retrieval cue. Cues referred to item function ('Doctors use it'), item class ('It's a tool'), or personal acquaintance ('I have one'). *(3) Asks for retrieval time.* Child asks for a retrieval delay ('Wait a second,...' 'I know it, let me see...'). *(4) Interrogates own retrieval.* Child overtly asks retrieval questions ('What *is* that?' 'What is that name?'). *(5) Affirms retrieval possibility.* Child states that he or she can retrieve the name ('I know that.' 'I know that name.'). *(6) Retrieval effort release.* Upon hearing the name in recognition, child indicates that effortful retrieval is now terminated ('That's what it was!' 'That's the one I was trying to think of!'). Rater reliability was 0.95 for coding these categories.

Did a positive feeling of knowing the name lead to increased later retrieval effort? Table III shows the data. At all ages significantly more ef-

Table III. Percentage of items receiving retrieval effort

	Grades		
	K	1	3
Feeling-of-knowing +	15	21	22
Feeling-of-knowing –	03	02	05

fort was directed to feeling-of-knowing + items, and almost no retrieval effort given to feeling-of-knowing – items.

This is not the only data of this sort. Research by *Lachman* et al. [1979] with adults shows similar results, as does a study by *Gruneburg and Monks* [1974]. In a different vein, *Posnansky* [1978] presented children with items to remember that were blocked in different sized categories. Before recall, she had some of the subjects estimate how large they thought the various categories were. During recall, she indexed search strategies. Consider for a moment your own possible actions in such a retrieval task. If you were recalling items in one category and could not quickly remember any more names, how long should you continue to search? One obvious strategy would be to search longer if you estimate there were many unrecalled items left in that category. On the other hand, you should quickly move to different categories if there were few or, especially, no unrecalled items left. *Posnansky* [1978] found that both kindergarteners and third graders exhibited this pattern of effort allocation in their responses. Importantly, effort allocation depended on the number of unrecalled items as based on each child's *judgment* of category size, not on true category size. Thus it was the metamemory assessments that were highly related to appropriate search effort.

The above studies concern allocation of retrieval effort; there are also investigations of study effort. *Bisanz* et al. [1978] presented first, third, fifth graders and college students with a list of paired associates to learn. The list was presented over a number of trials. After the first trial, when a cue was presented, a paired response was elicited *and* the subjects stated whether they judged their response had been correct or not. *Bisanz* et al.'s [1978] data showed that even kindergarteners could accurately discriminate between correct and incorrect items in these judgments. In addition, they presented evidence that, with age, this knowledge was used to allocate study time on subsequent trials. *Bisanz* et al.'s [1978] analysis is somewhat indirect since they had to infer study time apportionment from a measure of accuracy. But a study by *Masur* et al. [1973] showed that in a similar situation third graders, but not first graders, allocated future study effort on the basis of their estimates as to which items they had already sufficiently learned and which not.

As a final example, though I do not believe this exhausts the published literature, *Brown and Smilely* [1978] have presented data on the development of what amounts to various effort allocation strategies for remembering written text. A clear finding was that, with age, effort allocation comes to depend on the child's judgment of what is essential and what is not in the to-be-remembered material. Indeed all of the above studies show a clear link between metamemory and effort allocation. In some of these studies this link is shown even for the youngest children, in others it is absent in the youngest group but obviously develops thereafter.

I am not sure why the metamemory to performance link is so clear in these studies of effort allocation strategies. I can identify three possibilities all of which have implications for future research on the larger metamemory-memory question.

One possibility, consistent with the earlier discussion concerning methods, is that these studies of effort allocation are less like correlational research and more like manipulative experimental research. The child's metamemory judgments are manipulated – for example, he or she sees some items which provoke positive feeling-of-knowing judgments and also some which do not – then subsequent memory efforts are observed.

Another possibility is that the metamemory judgments in most (but not all) of these studies are of that one variety earlier called assessments of the current state of one's own memory. Perhaps, along the lines of *Flavell's* [1979] distinction between metacognitive knowledge and metacognitive experiences, these judgments have clearer experiential impact and, thus, more compelling behavioral implications for the subject.

There is a third possibility, and it is the one I favor at the moment. Just as there is a more informative level of metamemory to study – that of the child's integrated theory of memory – there exists a more informative level of memory strategy to be studying, at least in respect to metamemory's role. That is, stemming from the notion of general effort allocation strategies, we could be studying the child's memory development as a variety of decision making. Strategic effort allocation is one form of such a decision making process. If we conceive of the development of memory itself as the development of applied mnemonic decision making, then it may be more obvious how various sorts of knowledge, including metamemory, play a role in this process.

Conclusion

The two foci of this paper have been: What is metamemory, and what is its role? As I warned in advance, my discussion of these topics has been a personal one. It is personal in the following sense, captured in a quotation from *Klahr* [1978, p. 192]:

> 'One productive way to view the enterprise of theory construction is to characterize it as a search through a large problem space. Different theorists make different decisions about how to traverse the many paths available to them in constructing their theories and in deciding how to gather more information to help them get to the next state. As in the search of any complex problem space, there are some states from which further progress appears to be impossible. Others appear to have the potential for success... One proceeds through such problem spaces using a variety of scientific problem-solving strategies, heuristics, and rules of thumb.'

In short, this paper offers my view as to 'where we are' in understanding metamemory, and my hunches as to which future paths have great or small potential for successfully leading to advances in our understanding [*Wellman*, in press].

To summarize, first, what is metamemory? From the point of view of the investigator, metamemory is a cover term referring to a family of knowledge about memory and cognition. It should not be considered a precise theoretical construct but an ill-defined concept which usefully directs our attention and research to a distinctive aspect of memory behavior. Thus, its theoretical value lies not so much in the general construct, but that this distinctive perspective has the potential of yielding derivative theoretical constructs of precision and power.

Second, what is metamemory development the development of? For the child, it is the development of an intricately interrelated system of knowledge, a theory or theories of memory embedded within a larger theory of cognition, embedded within a larger theory of human behavior. At this point we know dismayingly little about metamemory from this point of view. These larger theories of memory can be investigated by assessing the child's integration of different memory facts, beliefs, or expectancies; they can be investigated by charting the child's naive understanding of certain theoretical notions central to psychological explanations of memory itself; they can be investigated by exploring the child's conception of the mental world in general, and conceptions of the relation and difference between mental and behavioral acts.[1]

Third, what role does metamemory play? There is no question but that some sorts of knowledge about memory figure strongly into some sorts of memory performances and that this changes with age. Exactly how, where, and when metamemory does and does not play what role is relatively uncharted territory. However, at least two paths for future exploration recommend themselves. First, the metamemory incorporated into studies of metamemory-memory relations should be the type just spoken of: assessments which try to capture the child's larger integrated notions of the array of explicit and implicit factors affecting memory. Second, the memory involved in such investigations could be fruitfully considered as applied mnemonic decision-making, especially decision making in regard to effort allocation. This may offer a model of mnemonic processes which more cogently captures the imprint of metamemory. To elaborate this suggestion somewhat, current research on attributional determinants of task performance provides a reasonable analogy for how to investigate the metamnemonic determinants of memory performance. In the attributional research [*Parsons*, in press] the person is seen as possessing a complex system of beliefs, knowledge, and expectancies about personal abilities and goals as well as task attributes and values. These interact in

[1] Richer knowledge of children's understanding of the mind and its place within human behavior is necessary for another line of research as well, the study of awareness. In studies of children's awareness of their mental processes an investigator collects independent evidence of the child's engaging in some mental process and then, typically, asks if he or she engaged in that process [*Nisbett and Wilson,* 1977]. Concordance of presence or absence of report with engagement or not in the process is taken as evidence of awareness. One problem, as philosophers point out [*Anscombe,* 1976], is that awareness must be understood as 'awareness under a description'. I am only aware of X under some description of X. If I am rehearsing items my awareness of my act may include, 'saying the names' and 'saying them over', but not 'rehearsing them', 'maintaining the items in short-term memory' or other descriptions. If told, for example, 'you were maintaining a trace of the items in some cortical resonance circuit' I could legitimately say, 'I was not aware I was doing that' while still being aware of what I was doing *under some description*. Thus, in investigating the development of awareness, children's developing descriptions of the mind and its processes play a crucial role. Answers to questions used as an index to awareness depend on awareness and on mental descriptions, that is, on larger theories and understanding of mental phenomena.

numerous ways to determine type of task engaged in, persistence on task, accepted level of performance, etc. In short, complex personal theories mediate task-relevant effort allocation. Indeed, given a broad definition of metacognition, this research is itself a demonstration of the influence of metacognition on performance.

References

Ajzen, I.; Fishbein, M.: Attitude-behavior relations: a theoretical analysis and review of empirical research. Psychol. Bull. *84:* 888–918 (1977).

Anscombe, G.E.M.: Intention; 2nd ed. (Cornell University Press, New York 1976).

Baker, L.; Brown, A.L.: Metacognitive skills of reading; in Pearson, Handbook of reading research (in press).

Bisanz, G.L.; Vesonder, G.T.; Voss, J.F.: Knowledge of one's own responding and the relation of such knowledge to learning. J. exp. Child Psychol. *25:* 116–128 (1978).

Brown, A.L.; Smilely, S.S.: The development of strategies for studying texts. Child Dev. *49:* 1076–1088 (1978).

Cavanaugh, J.C.; Borkowski, J.G.: Searching for metamemory-memory connections: a developmental study. Devl Psychol. *16:* 441–453 (1980).

Cavanaugh, J.C.; Perlmutter, M.: Metamemory: a critical examination. Child Dev. *53:* 11–28 (1982).

Cialdini, R.B.; Petty, R.E.; Cacioppo, J.T.: Attitude and attitude change. A. Rev. Psychol. *32:* 357–404 (1981).

Cook, T.D.; Campbell, D.T.: Quasi-experimentation: design and analysis issues for field settings (Rand McNally, Chicago 1979).

Fabricius, W.; Wellman, H.M.: Children's understanding of retrieval cue utilization Devl. Psychol. *19:* 15–21 (1983).

Flavell, J.H.: First discussant's comments: What is memory development the development of? Hum. Dev. *14:* 272–278 (1971).

Flavell, J.H.: Metacognitive development; in Scandura, Brainerd, Structural/process theories of complex behavior (Sitjoff & Nordhoff, Leyden 1978).

Flavell, J.H.: Metacognition and cognitive monitoring: a new area of cognitive-developmental inquiry. Am. Psychol. *34:* 906–911 (1979).

Flavell, J.H.; Friedrichs, A.G.; Hoyt, J.D.: Developmental changes in memorization processes. Cognitive Sci. *1:* 324–340 (1970).

Flavell, J.H.; Wellman, H.M.: Metamemory; in Kail, Hagen, Perspectives on the development of memory and cognition, pp. 3–33 (Erlbaum, Hillsdale 1977).

Gruneburg, M.M.; Monks, J.: Feeling of knowing and cued recall. Acta psychol. *38:* 251–265 (1974).

Hayes-Roth, B.; Hayes-Roth, F.: A cognitive model of planning. Cognitive Sci. *3:* 275–310 (1979).

Johnson, C.N.; Wellman, H.M.: Children's developing conceptions of the mind and brain. Child Dev. *53:* 222–234 (1982).

Klahr, D.: Rages over stages. Behavioral Brain Sci. *2:* 191–192 (1978).

Lachman, J.L.; Lachman, R.; Thronesbury, C.: Metamemory through the adult life span. Devl Psychol. *15:* 543–551 (1979).

Masur, E.F.; McIntyre, C.W.; Flavell, J.H.: Developmental changes in apportionment of study time among items in a multi-trial free recall task. J. exp. Child Psychol. *15:* 237–246 (1973).

Nisbett, R.E.; Wilson, T.D.: Telling more than we know: verbal reports on mental processes. Psychol. Rev. *84:* 231–259 (1977).

Paris, S.G.: Metacognitive development: children's regulation of problem solving skills. Proc. Annu. Meet. of the Midwestern Psychological Association, Chicago 1978.

Parsons, J.E.: Expectancies, values, and academic behaviors; in Spence, Assessing achievement (Freeman, San Francisco, in press).

Posnansky, C.J.: Age- and task-related differences in the use of category size information for retrieval of categorized items. J. exp. Child Psychol. *26:* 373–382 (1978).

Salatas, H.; Flavell, J.H.: Behavioral and metamnemonic indicators of strategic behaviors under remember instructions in first grade. Child Dev. *47:* 81–89 (1976).

Wellman, H.M.: Tip of the tongue and feeling of knowing experience: a developmental study of memory monitoring. Child Dev. *48:* 13–21 (1977).

Wellman, H.M.: Knowledge of the interaction of memory variables. Devl Psychol. *14:* 24–29 (1978).

Wellman, H.M.: A child's theory of mind: the development of conceptions of cognition; in Yussen, The growth of insight in the child (in press).

Wellman, H.M.; Collins, J.; Gleiberman, G.: Understanding the combination of memory variables: developing conceptions of memory limitations. Child Dev. *52:* 1313–1317 (1981).

Wicker, A.W.: Attitudes versus action: the relationship of verbal and overt behavioral responses to attitude objects. J. soc. Issues *25:* 41–78 (1969).

Wilensky, R.: Meta-planning: representing and using knowledge about planning in problem solving and natural language understanding. Cognitive Sci. *5:* 197–233 (1981).

Contr. hum. Dev., vol. 9, pp. 52–70 (Karger, Basel 1983)

Scripts and the Development of Memory

Katherine Nelson, Robyn Fivush, Judith Hudson, Joan Lucariello
City University of New York, New York, N.Y., USA

Much attention has been given in recent years to the effect of real world knowledge on the interpretation, comprehension and reconstruction of material in memory. This emphasis reflects a constructive, 'top-down', schematic view of comprehension and memory. Our work on children's scripts for real world events is directed toward understanding the structure and function of their real world knowledge, how it develops and how it affects cognitive processing, in particular, memory of various kinds. In this way we hope to shed light on the development of top-down processing. For example, where does the 'top' come from? Is it itself constructed bottom-up, or is it basic to comprehension and memory throughout the life span?

We suggest that there are two major relationships of script knowledge to the development of memory. First, most current theories of memory attribute an organizing function to the existing knowledge base that the individual brings to a memory task. This assumption was set forth originally and most persuasively by *Bartlett* [1932] and has been enthusiastically revitalized in recent years in terms of constructive theories of memory. In order to understand what happens when children try to remember something, given this assumption, it is necessary to understand the content and structure of their knowledge base. Note that we cannot specify this knowledge simply in terms of *logical* structures (such as the ability to make inferences or to classify) but we need to understand *what* children know and in what form it is stored. Nor is it enough to understand what they do *not* know, which has been the focus of so much research on the young child's mind, yielding a rich collection of deficiencies, but leaving us with an understanding that is as empty as the young child's mind is inferred to be.

Of course the assumption is widespread – even among those who deal with young children – that the knowledge base of the young child is disorganized, idiosyncratic, fragmented, and even amusing in its beliefs about the nature of reality, for example, that clouds and the moon are alive. These assumptions have been supported by previous research. For example, research on memory in young children focused on children's strategies for recalling categorically organized lists of words [see *Hagen* et al., 1975, for a review] generally concludes that children younger than about 7 years old are unable to organize their recall into taxonomic categories, but with increasing age, children become more efficient at organizing such material in memory.

Yet we know (at least, those who deal with young children feel they do) that children operate in the world with evident rich beliefs and attitudes. We need then a description of the knowledge base that can account for them. Recent theorists have argued that young children's knowledge is organized schematically rather than categorically [*Mandler,* in press]. Schemas are generaly described as spatially-temporally organized sets of expectations about what things will look like or the order in which events will occur. These expectations are organized in terms of a series of variables, or slots, which can be instantiated with greater or lesser degrees of probability by a range of values. Examples of schematically organized knowledge include scenes, stories and events.

The proposal that children's knowledge is organized around sets of expectations for familiar objects, people, places and events has several implications for how children remember. Schema models stress the dynamic and constructive use of schemas in organizing comprehension and memory. Because they act as unified bodies of knowledge, when particular schemas are activated, they automatically operate in a top-down, conceptually driven process to structure and give meaning to material by assigning values to the constituent variables. If a situation does not provide enough information to instantiate a variable, the values of the other variables as well as expectations about allowable and probable values can lead to the assignment of default values. Comprehension and recall of schematically organized material is therefore highly inferential in nature and can even produce distortions in memory.

Evidence for schematic organization of children's knowledge comes from studies demonstrating constructive processes in comprehension and memory. Research on how children remember and make inferences about related sentences [*Barclay and Reid,* 1974; *Bransford* et al., 1972; *Brans-*

ford and McCarrell, 1974; *Paris and Lindauer,* 1976, 1977; *Paris and Mahoney,* 1974; *Paris and Upton,* 1976], connected prose [*Brown,* 1976a; *Brown and French,* 1976], and pictures [*Brown,* 1976b] indicated that children can integrate semantically related material as unified wholes, make appropriate inferences, and tend to falsely recognize consistent but not presented material. Studies of children's recall for stories [*Mandler,* 1978; *Stein and Glenn,* 1979] showed that children recall simple stories remarkably well and organize their recall in the same way as adults. *Mandler* [1978] has argued that story recall is guided by a general story schema which specifies event categories or nodes, such as reactions, goal-path attempts and outcomes. Both children and adults tend to recall sentences from each of the major story nodes. Further, when stories are presented in a scrambled order, children and adults restructure the material to conform to the canonical order even when asked to recall the story in the presented order. These findings suggest that story schemas automatically guide retrieval of story narratives. It seems, then, that children do operate with organized knowledge about their world which they can use in memory tasks when the material to be remembered matches the organization of the knowledge base.

The second reason that the content of children's knowledge is important is that it is a sure guide to what children will naturally remember. As we all know, children below the age of 7 or 8 are notoriously poor at remembering items in memory tasks such as the contents of a set of objects, pictures or words, word lists, and so on. Recent studies have attempted to show that young children remember better when the material to be remembered is embedded in a more meaningful or naturalistic context. When preschool children are engaged in a meaningful activity, they can remember a list of words [*Istomina,* 1975], recall the spatial location of various objects [*Myers, Perlmutter and Sophian,* as reported in *Myers and Perlmutter,* 1978], and even recall the location of a hidden object after several days delay [*DeLoache,* 1980; *DeLoache and Brown,* 1979]. This is in accord with the Soviet view of involuntary memory [see *Meacham,* 1972, 1977, for a review]. Material which is related to the individual's activity or goals will be automatically remembered because the ongoing activity provides a meaningful context or organization for subsequent recall.

The study of the natural knowledge base allows us to go beyond the study of naturalistic memory *tasks* and to discover what children naturally remember from a given experience: How do they allocate their memory functions in everyday life? How much and what sorts of things get stored and in what form? Recent studies [*Ratner,* 1980; *Todd and Perlmutter,* 1980] suggest that this is a rich and informative area of inquiry. By studying these aspects of the young child's mind, we hope to shed light, not only on the developing short-term memory system, but on such intriguing questions as why the long-term episodic memory system – i.e. autobiographical memory – appears to become permanently activated only after the age of 3 or 4 years.

Here we will report three types of studies that are relevant to these issues and that have revealed some answers to previously unasked questions about young children's thought: First, what do children remember about events that they experience and what form does the memory take? Second, how specifically does prior knowledge about events determine what will be remembered about a new episode, or the report of a new episode in story form? Third, how does the child's understanding of events in the real world affect the way in which memory tasks are approached?

The framework that we have used in this work is based on the script model developed by *Schank and Abelson* [1977]. Their analysis of the structure of events and the type of knowledge both people and computers must have to interpret narratives about events provided us with a starting point. Subsequent work has convinced us that scripts are indeed a basic form of knowledge representation for young children.

In brief, the script is a schematic organization that represents an event structure based on experience in the real world. It is organized in terms of temporal and causal relations between its component acts. Each script has a central or goal act and specifies which acts and items are required and which are optional or variable over contexts. For optional acts or items there are default values, stating what is to be expected in the usual case if the item is not specified in a particular instance. Thus, with a script representation of, say, eating at a restaurant, one can predict that there will be a waiter or waitress, a menu, food will be brought to the table, there will be a bill presented at the end, and so on. Optionally one may be expected to pay the waiter or the cashier at the door. In the fast food script, payment occurs before eating. Thus, different paths must be set up on the basis of different experiences with the same general situation. It is important to note that scripts are a form of general and not specific knowledge. Thus, they are one form of what *Piaget* termed 'memory in the broad sense' [*Piaget and Inhelder,* 1973]. Yet, paradoxically, they appear to be also a form of episodic memory in that they are derived from the experience of episodes in the real world. In this report we will consider script representations in relation to both general and specific memory, since scripts are both a form of general memory and influence what specific information is retained in episodic memory.

The Structure of Children's Script Memory

How are scripts formed and how do they develop? Can structural characteristics of scripts be identified and are they reliably extracted from the situation by young children? These were the first questions that we addressed [*Gruendel,* 1980; *Nelson,* 1978a, 1981; *Nelson and Gruendel,* 1979, 1980, 1981]. To answer them, we carried out a series of studies that required children to report on some very familiar and personally meaningful events as well as some relatively unfamiliar and personally uninvolving events; to act out events with props; to arrange pictures in sequence and tell stories about them [*Fivush and Nelson,* in preparation; *Nelson and Gruendel,* 1981].

Although most of our work thus far has involved verbalization of script knowledge, we do not consider that the verbalization reflects all the child knows about a script nor does it indicate that script knowledge is itself verbal. It is, however, convenient and also somewhat surprising that even very young children find it natural to talk about their event knowledge, and we assume that what they tell us about it has some significance; that is, there is a reason for choosing what to say and how to say it. Indeed, our data show that this assumption is correct.

Before claiming that children have knowledge in the form of scripts (i.e. temporal-causal chains of actions organized around a goal), we need to ask what the alternatives are – what else could they have? For example, they might have stimulus-response (s-r) chains where one action leads to another, but there is no overall organizing structure. This has been a common view of young children's minds over the years. According to this model, if one started a child reporting on dinner at eating dessert he or she should have difficulty in *reversing* to the prior act of cooking dinner or leaping forward to the much later act of going to bed. Another very common view of the young child's mind is that he or she might have stored quite unordered bits and pieces of knowledge of a domain. For example, a child might know that he or she had chocolate ice cream and played pin-the-tail-on-the-donkey at a birthday party, but not know what the general *structure* of a birthday party is. A third way that children's knowledge might be organized is according to different principles – association structures specifying what goes with what, for example, so that if one asked about getting dressed a child might tell you about all the different kinds of shirts or pants or dresses he or she has. Or, if similarity was the operating principle, the response might be things that look like each other. A fourth possibility is memory for a particular *episode* or a collection of episodes that is organized but quite *specific* in its details. Now these last two types of organization are not mutually exclusive with the generalized *script* structure. We do not claim that the human mind – even the young human mind – is confined to one kind of organizing principle. However, in previous research it has often been difficult to find *any* conceptual organization of young children's knowledge beyond the organization provided by the immediate perceptual context. It has usually been concluded, therefore, that young children are conceptually inept or deficient.

Considering these alternatives to scripts, the evidence is very strong that children *do* have generalized event scripts, that is, they organize their knowledge of familiar events according to generalized temporal and causal sequences of acts. Consider the youngest child (aged just 3 years) that we have interviewed within the frame of asking, 'What happens when you do x?'

Making cookies: 'Well, you bake them and you eat them.'
Birthday party: 'You cook a cake and eat it.'
Restaurant: 'You eat and then you go somewhere.'
Grocery shopping: 'You buy things and then you go home.'
Getting dressed: 'You put on your clothes and then you have breakfast.'

Each of this child's answers links two acts basic to the event, including a central or goal act, by the temporal linking terms 'and' or 'and then'. In each case the order is correct. Note that there was no intrusion of idiosyncratic or unordered material, or simple episodic reporting. These responses are not simple verbalizations of s-r chains, since the particular acts that are linked are not necessarily closely linked in time, and they are not elicited by a prior action but by an organizing term or script *header*: you have a *party* or go to a *restaurant*. Moreover, and this is important, they do not refer to elemental actions but whole events: 'You *bake* them' involves innumerable steps, usually steps carried out by someone else. The child's ability to subsume this activity under a single *general* term is significant.

Indeed, these reports, like most that we have gathered, are at a very high level of generality – here there are no particulars mentioned at all.

Further evidence of the generality of children's scripts is in the language in which the reports are phrased. Children tend to use very general terms such as 'you eat' or 'you play' rather than 'you swing' or 'you ride bikes'. These specifications leave open many possibilities for inserting variable slot fillers. It is of considerable interest that even the youngest children – 3- and 4-year-olds – found the 'timeless event' present tense form of the verb (e.g., 'eat' instead of 'ate') and the general use of 'you' and 'we' to be natural forms for reporting in this task. These forms have rarely been reported before in ordinary discourse by young children. We believe their use indicates a general level of knowledge that has not been tapped in previous research.

Let us try to clarify what we think is the significance of the generality of young children's scripts. It goes against the notion that children are drawing on a store of accumulated episodes that are remembered in some detail and from which a more abstract prototypical structure is later derived. They are already *categorical* in the sense of being general with examples of what can fill slots [*Abelson*, 1976]. Although most of our data are based on scripts that are already highly familiar to children, we have some data for events that are not, for example, day-care scripts from children in their first week at the day-care center and fire drill scripts from children who have experienced only one fire drill. We find the same form – general and skeletal – in these as in more familiar events. Thus, we believe that the script report is not being generated from the specific memory of a single particular experience but rather from a structure that is already generalized, that has open slots for variable roles and objects such as particular teachers, foods and games. It is our strong hypothesis that young children's knowledge of event structures is *generalized from the outset*; that is, that the *first* experience of an event leads to an expectation that further experiences of the kind will contain the same basic elements and relationships and an *open* structure is set up for this purpose.

This speculation is highly relevant to the question of how scripts develop, both in the short run and over time, as cognitive growth proceeds. In the studies we have done thus far, we have found that older children, say, 5- or 8-year-olds, compared to 3- and 4-year-olds, give longer scripts, remember more, use more complex language and report more conditional or alternative paths. For example, when asked to tell about restaurants, they will say, 'if we go to McDonald's' or 'when we go to Macy's'. That is to be expected on the basis of their greater general cognitive and linguistic maturity. But we have *not* found that there is a change in the basic *structure* of the script, at least from ages 3 to 8. 3-year-olds, as we indicated before, structure their knowledge using the same *generalized temporal-causal sequences* that older children do. They leave out more details and their reports are often exceedingly short and skeletal; however, the basics are there.

Effects of Script Structure on Constructive Memory

We have recently conducted a series of studies aimed at examining more closely the structural characteristics of children's scripts as brought to bear on different types of memory tasks. We expected that the script structure would influence the selection of material remembered as well as the organization of children's recall. In particular, we predicted: (1) The temporal-causal structure of the script should act as a powerful organizer in recall. (2) The general level of the script should be reflected in the selection of material recalled as well as in constructive inferences in recall. (3) Children should be consistent over time in what they remember if recall is guided by a relatively permanent representation.

One area of investigation has been the role of goals in organizing children's scripts. Because preschool children inevitably experience activities from a different perspective than adults, it seemed plausible that their goals for events could be quite different from ours. For example, going to a restaurant seems to be a very boring activity for young children. Unlike most adults, they have a hard time getting into the spirit of it. But according to theory, goals are supposed to motivate script formation. How sensitive are children to the goals around which scripts are presumed to be organized? If they do not share our goals, do they have their own? Do goals really make a difference to script formation?

In a recent experiment designed and carried out by *Hudson* [1981] to explore these questions, we presented children with stories about two events – birthday party and making cookies. In one condition, the goal statement was explicitly stated at the outset, while in the other there was no goal statement but a neutral 'setting' statement, for example, 'George and his mother were in the kitchen', rather than 'George and his mother decided to make cookies'. Pre-school children and first graders heard brief stories about the events and were asked to retell them, both immediately and again after the lapse of a day. There was no difference at either time between the goal and goalless stories in amount of recall, and almost all children were able to state the goal at the conclusion of the story. Indeed, half the preschoolers added a goal statement to their recall. That is, children inferred the goal from the sequence of events even when it was not stated explicitly. On the basis of this experiment then, it appears that our original suspicion that goals were not as *apparent* to children as to adults was in error. On the other hand, even if children build their scripts around goals just as adults do, it may still be the case that their goals differ from adults' in particular instances. This question has not received a definitive answer as yet; more research in this area is needed.

This study also provided evidence of effects of script structure on the temporal-causal organization of children's recall. In addition to the goalless story condition, we presented the stories in a misordered form that violated the canonical order of events. For example, the birthday party story stated that children brought presents at the end rather than the beginning. Research with adults [*Bower* et al., 1979] found a tendency to *repair* misordered narratives in recall in the directions of the canonical script. Our results showed similar effects of script structure on recall; children usually omitted one or both of the actions that were out of order in their recall; or they moved an act to its correct position in the temporal-causal sequence, (e.g., making the presents at the end be party favors that the guests took home). These repairs are similar to those observed in recall for stories by older children and adults when a story schema is deformed [*Mandler and DeForest*, 1979; *Stein and Glenn*, 1979].

In a study previously reported by *McCartney and Nelson* [1981] we also found effects of scripts on memory for stories in the *selection* of parts recalled. Children 5 and 7 years old selectively remembered the main acts (rather than the details) of a story about a familiar event (dinner and bedtime). These selections and repairs in recall indicate the influence of well-structured scripts on memory in very young children.

Our experimental research, so far, supports our more naturalistic data. We have found further evidence that children structure their knowledge in the form of generalized temporal-causal sequences of actions which not only direct the way in which they talk about events, but influence how they approach memory tasks. We are also beginning to explore some of the ways in which these representations are built up through experience as well as developmental changes in the effects of script structures on the organization of the knowledge base.

Scripts and Memory for Novel Events

How does the existence of a script affect what a child will remember of a new experience? There is a certain amount of ambiguity and recursion here. Given the general assumption that no one faces any experience de novo, but always structures understanding in the light of prior schemas or other organizing structures, the question of what is novel becomes a highly subjective and ambiguous one. It has given us pause in constructing our research methods. Novelty for a child within our model can range from a slight variation on a highly familiar event, being presented with a new food for dinner, for example, to an experience that simply has no counterpart in terms of previous life experience, for example, going to the circus for the first time, or the first day at school (if there has been no pre-school experience). For most of us, most of the time, there is no totally novel experience. (Even the first moon-walkers were well rehearsed for the experience.) Thus, we assume that any experience is organized in terms of some similar experience: the script that fits most closely. For example, going to the circus might be seen as a variation on the outing script that includes going to the zoo or to an amusement park.

Given that this is the case, how will the prior script affect the memory for the new experience and, conversely, how will the new experience affect the old script? The latter question is currently under study in terms of script development. Let us consider the first question in light of our present research findings.

In one study (carried out by *Hudson and Morse*), 3- and 5-year-old children were asked on one occasion the general question, 'What happens when you have dinner at home (or snack at camp)?' and on another occasion the specific question, 'What happened one time (or yesterday)?' There was a clear differentiation between the use of the general present tense for the general account and the past tense for the specific account. Moreover, there was also a greater use of particular terms, that is, slot fillers, in the specific accounts. Thus, it was clear that the children were distinguishing between the two questions.

For example:

General: 'We go to snack and then. ... we get up, finish snack, have naptime, get into our bathing suits and swim' (4.10). 'We eat dinner. We go to bed' (5.1). 'After dinner we have dessert. We get dessert. We go to bed' (2.9).

Specific: 'Oh we ate, I think we ate snack in the library. We had saltines, double saltines and milk. And that's all' (4.10). 'I had apple juice and grape juice. Some grape juice at one table and other juice at the other table' (3.7). 'I ate a piece of salami with a piece of bread ... After dinner I got washed and I got ready for Disney World' (3.4).

Surprisingly, the young children found it *more* difficult to give a specific memory than they did a general account, regardless of order. In general, there were more children who gave no responses, and accounts were briefer when they were asked the specific than the general question. Our tentative explanation for this finding is that the general script actually *interferes with* the memory of a specific episode; for a routine event like eating dinner, each new episode is absorbed by the script structure. While younger children seem not to hold on to any specific variations, older children and adults might have developed mechanisms whereby some episodes become tagged as memorable in themselves, in this way developing an autobiographical memory.

However, there is another side to be considered. We have also found that when a child reports a unique experience, such as going to the circus, the reports may be long and detailed. This accords with the findings of *Todd and Perlmutter* [1980] who were able to elicit many specific episodic memories from 3- and 4-year-old children. One way of resolving this apparent contradiction, i.e. that the same novel experience may be held in memory in either general, skeletal or a specific, detailed form, is to assume that there are two different long-term memory processes, one for general knowledge and one for specific memories which produces autobiographical memory. The question then is, what is the relation between the two with respect to any given memory and also, and most intriguingly, with respect to the development of the memory system as a whole. In regard to the latter, it is interesting to note that autobiographical memories do not become established until about the age of three. This fact is of considerable interest to the theory of scripts and their development.

A script for a familiar event may provide a framework for remembering what happens in general (allowing prediction) as well as what happened on one particular occasion. However, this framework may have several other effects, for example, instead of remembering the specific event the episode may become *fused* into the general script so that it is no longer remembered as a particular episode, as we have found.

On the other hand, aspects of several different experiences may also become *confused* with each other. The notion of slot fillers and general categories may help to make clear the differences between these effects. A script is basically a framework that specifies at the most general level what takes place in a situation of a certain type. What happens at a restaurant? One orders, eats, pays and leaves. What and how to order, what and how to eat, who serves, whom to pay, where to go when leaving are all *variables* that fill certain slots in the script. The specific items that occur on particular occasions we call *slot fillers*. Thus, the hamburger eaten at McDonald's or the filet mignon at The Four Seasons are both slot-fillers. Now two different things may happen to the details of a particular experience. First, one may lose or fuse the details in the general script. One may know that one went to McDonald's on the way to skiing in Vermont but not remember anything further about the particular episode. It has become fused. However, one can *reconstruct* it through the script, using the script's default values or optional fillers in place of or to retrieve known slot fillers. Thus, one might be able to report: 'I had a hamburger and a large coke.'

On the other hand, different episodes may be *confused* with each other. For example, one may remember having a milkshake instead of a coke on a particular occasion. Both are appropriate slot fillers for the general script but only one is appropriate for the particular remembered occasion. *Neisser* [1981] has recently reported very similar effects in his analysis of the confusions and fusions by John Dean's memory for the details of the Watergate Coverup. He has introduced the notion of a 'repisode' for the report of a purported episode that is actually based on similar repeated experiences and in which details may be lost or confused.

A frequent occasion where fusion (rather than confusion) appears to operate is for the first experience of an event that later becomes routine. Some people remember their first day at school or on a new job in some detail, but it is surprising how many do not. In examining the early autobiographical memories of adults (based on our pilot work and review of older research), it is striking how many are of mild deviations from a routine – neither memories of a first experience nor of a strikingly novel one. Children's accounts seem to bear this out – they seem to need to build up a script before they can differentiate the somewhat novel event that is worth remembering for its own sake. At the beginning, the experiences fuse together.

For example, *Fivush* [in preparation] found that kindergarteners interviewed on the second day of school had difficulty recalling what they had done on the first day of school although they already had very general and skeletal school scripts. Two months later they had much more elaborate scripts but most were still unable to remember many specific happenings in that setting in the recent past.

In our seminar on memory development a few years ago, we carried through a replication of sorts of the autobiographical memory study that *Linton* [1975, 1979] has reported. The participants kept a record of what they believed would be memorable events each day during the course of the semester, writing cues on the front of a 7.62 × 12.7 cm card and a more complete description of the event on the back. At the end of the semester, a sample of the cards was selected and memory for the episodes was tested. There was a very systematic relation between the frequency of the type of episode recorded (high-frequency events being those such as attending class, going to the movies, etc.) and the difficulty of remembering it. Frequent events were often forgotten entirely – fused, that is, with their general scripts. Confusions, of course, are more difficult to identify in this paradigm, since inaccurate autobiographical memories are in most cases indistinguishable from accurate ones. The frequency effect we found replicates that reported by *Linton* [1979].

Thus, at least four effects of a prior script on memory for new experiences or narratives about such events have been identified and have been found to operate for children as young as 3. They are *fusion, confusion, selection* and *repair*. It is worth noting that, whenever we have found age differences in the extent to which these effects operate, they have been greater for younger than older children. That is, younger children appear to be *more* affected by the canonical script than older children are.

Scripts and Categorical Organization in Memory

The most widely studied paradigm in memory literature is no doubt that of free recall for lists of words. A study by *Lucariello and Nelson* [1982] used that paradigm to assess the effects of scripts on memory.

Many developmental and cross-cultural experiments have compared children's organization and memory for lists of taxonomically related words with those composed of presumably unrelated words. Although some effects have been positive, even for very young children [*Myers and Perlmutter*, 1978; *Rossi and Rossi*, 1965], most have been negative. Children below about age 8 benefit little from having related lists and do not reorder the lists in recall into clusters of related words as adults do [*Hagen* et al., 1975]. These results have been used to support the argument that young children do not understand or use hierarchical relations such as those reflected in taxonomic categories. However, there are many indications from psycholinguistic research [*Anglin*, 1977; *Nelson*, 1974, 1978b] that children can use and understand categorical relations in their natural speech even if they do not utilize them in memory. Indeed, it seems that all categories that have been suggested as ones that a young child might understand exist in the child's world as natural groupings of some sort.

Most category members used with young children that are found in spatial groups are also experienced in script frameworks. They occur as slot fillers in different eating, dressing, playing, scripts. This observation lay behind our recall study. If scripts are important to the formation of hierarchical categories, we believed that we should be able to manipulate their use in recall lists by varying the script relations contained therein.

For this experiment, then, we constructed two recall lists as follows: We first elicited lists of words from pre-schoolers in the categories of clothes, food and animals by questioning them about objects associated with a single action in a given script. Within the clothes category we asked children to tell us clothes they put on in the morning, those they wore outside and clothes they wore to bed. Within the animal category we asked for zoo, pet and farm animals, and within the food category we asked for breakfast, lunch and dessert foods. Next we took the most frequently mentioned response for each subcategory question and composed a taxonomic, hierarchical, context-free list of three each of animals, food and clothes. The script-based list was composed of the three most frequent responses in each of the following subcategories: zoo animals, lunch foods, and clothes you put on in the morning.

Two groups of pre-school children were presented with the taxonomic list in either a free or constrained recall condition using taxonomic cues such as 'all the animals on the list'. Two groups received the slot-filler list in the same two conditions. In addition, the slot-filler list was used in a script-cue condition in which children were asked to tell all the things they could eat for lunch, put on in the morning, or see at the zoo. The first four conditions compare the effect of the composition of the categories from 1 or 3 different scripts while the last two compare the effect of taxonomic or script cues on recall of the same (script-derived) list.

The results are straightforward. Recall was significantly higher for the slot-filler list, in comparison to the hierarchical context-free list, in both free and constrained recall conditions. Moreover, for free recall, clustering was significantly higher for the slot-filler list. The highest level of recall was found for the slot-filler list in the script-cue condition, indicating the salience of cues that reflect the basis on which categories are initially formed. Thus, our present evidence supports the hypothesis that not only do scripts provide a convenient memory structure, but they also serve to generate more abstract forms of memory organization, such as taxonomic categories that are useful in memorizing tasks as well as in other cognitive activities.

General Discussion

Two general findings have emerged from the research that we have reported here: (1) scripts for familiar events are a powerful form of general knowledge organization; and (2) specific or episodic memory is influenced by script structures through transformations of the input to fit canonical structures as well as through confusions of slot-fillers or through fusion of acts.

At this point we would like to consider what the implications of these findings are for our general understanding of memory and its development. First, it appears that we need to posit two interacting natural memory processes, one that extracts general structure and one that codes specific information. Together they produce the general schema with optional slot-fillers and paths. The first provides the structure, frame, gist or schema of an event (or narrative); the second provides the alternative particulars and their probability of occurring in the context of other particulars. These two processes can produce a reliable knowledge base useful for predicting, for guiding action, for making inferences. However, in themselves they do *not* provide a mechanism for remembering the totality of a specific episode: the dramatic sequence of a particular party, the plot of a particular movie, or a particular class or laboratory experience. It is our thesis that the gist structure and the probable alternative details are established in development before the ability to recall a whole specific event. It is the latter that appears as autobiographical memory at about the age of 3, 4 or even as late as 8 or 10 years for some individuals. As *Neisser* [1981] suggests, this type of memory may depend upon the use of rehearsal, to self or others. This is an intriguing suggestion that fits the developmental data well. However, the first two facets, the general frame and the optional particulars, appear to be well-developed even in very young children.

Thus, prior to the establishment of an autobiographical memory stream, the memory system is already devouring experience by its script formation and elaboration devices. Moreover, the script structure appears to provide a natural framework within which more categorical structures can be derived.

Through the study of young children's event representations and their use, we have identified areas of functioning in which children appear to be more competent than they have usually been said to be. We have shown that their memories are not jumbled and fragmented but highly organized and are used to organize new experiences. However, lest we be accused of suggesting that the 3-year-old is as competent as the 10-year-old, we need to provide some brief discussion of the limitations as well as the strengths of this kind of organization.

As has been suggested elsewhere [*Nelson and Gruendel*, 1981], the generalized event representation that emerges as a script provides for the young child a context within which to understand real-life episodes, both novel and routine. Young children appear to rely on their scripts for understanding even more than older children do. In every case where age differences have been found in our studies, they show younger children to remember according to a canonical script more than older children. To what extent can we say then that young children are employing such sophisticated processes as logical inference, reconstructive sequencing and other characteristics of constructive memory?

The research reviewed here suggests that pre-school children's productions do display characteristics that would lead us to infer these processes. For example, they infer the goal in a goalless story and repair incorrect temporal sequences. However, it may be that the very power of script representations lies in their capacity to make logical inferences and causal *reasoning* unnecessary; i.e. when the child enters an experience or hears a narrative, he or she may simply 'plug in' so to speak to an old script. The script representation itself then provides the causal chain and the missing parts. What looks like high-powered reasoning is actually the result of having a well-structured mapping available. It is true that the child infers on the basis of the script, but it need not be a logical inference, rather, a *representational* one. This speculation can account for the difficulty that young children have when faced with unfamiliar or abstract materials or tasks. While they are apparently good at abstracting and representing causal sequences based on their own experiences, and using these representations to predict, interpret, and act, there is little evidence that they can manipulate elements that are not personally meaningful in the same way.

We have suggested previously [*Nelson*, 1981] that the script representation provides a spatiotemporal context for interpreting experience. That is, the child is not necessarily tied to the immediate real-world context although he or she may be bound to a schematic representation of similar previously experienced contexts. But this mental representation may itself be as restricting – in terms of possible interpretations of events – as any constraint in the real world.

We assume that an important aspect of cognitive development is the increasing distancing of the child from familiar personal experience and the increasing ability to perform in domains that are free of spatiotemporal context, external or internal. This view of development suggests caution in the interpretation of the performance by somewhat older children as well as younger. We believe that basic script representations can provide the support for more abstract cognitive organizations as well as the basis for making inference-like statements. We also believe that this kind of performance may lead toward more abstract reasoning in less familiar situations. However, 'reasoning,' 'inferencing' and 'constructing' in highly familiar situations cannot be taken as evidence for logical or reasoning abilities unless it can be shown that the representation itself did not provide the answers.

There is nothing in this statement that is meant to denigrate the powerful achievements of the pre-school child. They appear to use the same kinds of representational structures that we do in many of the same ways. We only want to emphasize that reliance on these structures may give the appearance of greater competence than they actually posses and that we need to balance our assessment of their achievements with a caution about the interpretation of their performance in restricted contexts.

References

Abelson, R.P.: Script processing in attitude formation and decision making; in Carroll, Payne, Cognition and social behavior, pp. 33–45 (Erlbaum, Hillsdale 1976).

Anglin, J.: Word, object and conceptual development (Norton, New York 1977).

Barclay, J.R.; Reid, M.: Semantic integration in children's recall of discourse. Devl Psychol. *10:* 277–281 (1974).

Bartlett, F.C.: Remembering: a study in experimental and social psychology (Cambridge, New York 1932).

Bower, G.H.; Black, J.B.; Turner, T.T.: Scripts in memory for texts. Cognitive Psychol. *11:* 177–220 (1979).

Bransford, J.D.; Barclay, J.D.; Franks, J.J.: Sentence memory: a constructive vs. interpretive approach. Cognitive Psychol. *3:* 193–209 (1972).

Bransford, J.D.; McCarrell, N.S.: A sketch of a cognitive approach to comprehension; in Weiner, Palermo, Cognition and the symbolic process, pp. 189–229 (Erlbaum, Hillsdale 1974).

Brown, A.L.: Semantic integration in children's reconstruction of narrative sequences. Cognitive Psychol. *8:* 247–262 (1976a).

Brown, A.L.: The construction of temporal succession by preoperational children; in Pick, Minnesota Symp. on Child Psychology, vol. 10, pp. 28–83 (University of Minnesota, Minneapolis 1976b).

Brown, A.L.; French, L.A.: Construction and regeneration of logical sequences using causes and consequences. Child Dev. *47:* 930–940 (1976).

DeLoache, J.: Naturalistic studies of memory for object location in very young children; in Perlmutter, Children's memory: new directions for child development, No. 10 (Jossey-Bass, San Francisco 1980).

DeLoache, J.; Brown, A.L.: Looking for big bird: studies of memory in very young children. Lab. compar. Hum. Cognit. Newsl. *1:* 4 (1979).

Fivush, R.: Learning about school: the development of kindergartener's school scripts; diss., New York (1982).

Fivush, R.; Nelson, K.: Naturalistic and experimental assessment of children's knowledge of event sequences (in preparation).

Gruendel, J.M.: Scripts and stories: a study of children's event narratives; unpublished doct. diss., Yale (1980).

Hagen, J.W.; Jongeward, R.H.; Kail, R.V.: Cognitive perspectives on the development of memory; in Reese, Advances in child development and behavior, vol. 10, pp. 57–101 (Academic Press, New York 1975).

Hudson, J.: Effects of script structure on children's story recall. Proc. Am. Psychological Association Meet., Los Angeles 1981.

Istomina, Z.M.: The development of involuntary memory in preschool age children. Soviet Psychol. *13(4):* 5–64 (1975).

Linton, M.: Memory for real-world events; in Norman, Rummelhart, LNR Research Group, Explorations in cognition, pp. 376–404 (Freeman, San Francisco 1975).

Linton, M.: Cueing events in adults' and children's autobiographical memory. Proc. Am. Psychological Association Meet., New York 1979.

Lucariello, J.; Nelson, K.: Context and categories in young children's memory. Proc. Southeastern Conf. on Development, Baltimore 1982.

Mandler, J.M.: A code in the node. Discourse Processes *1:* 14–35 (1978).

Mandler, J.M.: Representation; in Flavell, Markman, Cognitive development, vol. 2 of Mussen, Carmichael's Manual of Child Psychology (Wiley, New York, in press).

Mandler, J.M.; DeForest, M.: Is there more than one way to recall a story? Child Dev. *50:* 886–889 (1979).

McCartney, K.; Nelson, K.: Children's use of scripts in story recall. Discourse Processes *4:* 59–70 (1981).

Meacham, J.A.: The development of memory abilities in the individual and society. Hum. Dev. *15:* 205–228 (1972).

Meacham, J.A.: Soviet investigations of memory development; in Kail, Hagen, Perspectives on the development of memory and cognition, pp. 273–295 (Erlbaum, Hillsdale 1977).

Myers, N.A.; Perlmutter, M.: Memory in the years 2 to 5; in Ornstein, Memory development in children, pp. 191–218 (Erlbaum, Hillsdale 1978).

Neisser, U.: John Dean's memory: a case study. Cognition *9:* 1–22 (1981).

Nelson, K.: Variations in children's concepts by age and category. Child Dev. *45:* 577–584 (1974).

Nelson, K.: How young children represent knowledge of their world in and out of language; in Siegler, Children's thinking: What develops?, pp. 255–273 (Erlbaum, Hillsdale 1978a).

Nelson, K.: Semantic development and the development of semantic memory; in Nelson, Children's language, vol. 1, pp. 39–80 (Gardner Press, New York 1978b).

Nelson, K.: Social cognition in a script framework; in Ross, Flavell, The development of social cognition in childhood (Cambridge University Press, New York 1981).

Nelson, K.; Gruendel, J.M.: From personal episode to social script: two dimensions in the development of event knowledge. Proc. Meet. of the Society for Research in Child Development, San Francisco 1979.

Nelson, K.; Gruendel, J.M.: At morning it's lunchtime: a scriptal view of children's dialogues. Discourse Processes *2:* 73–94 (1980).

Nelson, K.; Gruendel, J.M.: Generalized event representations: basic building blocks of cognitive development; in Brown, Lamb, Advances in developmental psychology, vol. 1, pp. 131–138 (Erlbaum, Hillsdale 1981).

Paris, S.G.; Lindauer, B.K.: The role of inference in children's comprehension and memory for sentences. Cognitive Psychol. *8:* 217–227 (1976).

Paris, S.G.; Lindauer, B.K.: Constructive aspects of children's comprehension and memory; in Kail, Hagen, Perspectives on the development of memory and cognition, pp. 35–60 (Erlbaum, Hillsdale 1977).

Paris, S.G.; Mahoney, G.J.: Cognitive integration in children's memory for sentences and pictures. Child Dev. *45:* 633–642 (1974).

Paris, S.G.; Upton, L.R.: Children's memory for inferential relations in prose. Child Dev. *47:* 660–668 (1976).

Piaget, J.; Inhelder, B.: Memory and intelligence (Basic Books, New York 1973).

Ratner, H.H.: The role of social context in memory development; in Perlmutter, Children's memory: new directions for child development, No. 10 (Jossey-Bass, San Francisco 1980).

Rossi, E.L.; Rossi, S.I.: Concept utilization, serial order and recall in nursery-school children. Child Dev. *36:* 771–778 (1965).

Schank, R.C.; Abelson, R.P.: Scripts, plans, goals and understanding (Erlbaum, Hillsdale 1977).

Stein, N.A.; Glenn, C.: An analysis of story comprehension; in Freedle, New directions in discourse processing, vol. 2 (Ablex, Norwood 1979).

Todd, C.M.; Perlmutter, M.: Reality recalled by preschool children; in Perlmutter, Children's memory: new directions for child development, No. 10 (Jossey-Bass, San Francisco 1980).

Contr. hum. Dev., vol. 9, pp. 71–107 (Karger, Basel 1983)

A Learning Framework for Development

Michelene T.H. Chi, Ernest T. Rees
University of Pittsburgh, Pittsburgh, Pa., USA

Recently, developmental psychologists have become more aware of the importance of knowledge in the phenomena they have observed. Although traditional Piagetians often discussed knowledge, they tended to refer more to abstract abilities and logical structures. When a child acquired conservation, a concept was acquired which, while it could certainly be called knowledge, was knowledge on a plane above, and separate from, the plane of everyday factual knowledge. Just a decade ago, in the 1971 symposium on memory development, only two of the six papers made reference to knowledge. In *Corsini's* [1971, p. 231] paper, the word knowledge was not explicitly used; however, he did say, 'In a very real sense, what is coded ... is determined by the existing cognitive store at any given point in time'. In his conclusion, though, he did not place a great emphasis on 'the development of a general information base' [p. 234], listing it only as one of five possible sources of development. *Flavell* [1971, p. 273], in his discussion, did say directly, 'It has long been clear that what we know... determines what and how we perceive, or speak, or imagine, or problem solve, or predict; it is now becoming equally clear that all that knowledge ... shape(s) what and how we learn and remember'. At the conclusion of his paper, however, he referred to knowledge in the more narrow context of knowledge about storage and retrieval operations, or metaknowledge.

The fact that knowledge acquisition has not been popular as the major source of development stems from a variety of observations that seem to indicate a limitation that cannot be overcome simply by imbuing the child with more knowledge. However, more careful recent work has shown the importance of the knowledge a child already possesses to the ability to learn what is being taught. Just as it is not wise to take a course in school without the prerequisites, it is equally unwise to try to teach children knowledge for which they are unprepared. Recent advances made by developmental researchers in pinpointing exactly what knowledge a child is bringing to a task, and by researchers in cognitive science in modeling human memory and learning, necessitate that developmentalists take another look at exactly how much of development is really due to learning rather than to some kind of change in innate physical or mental structures.

Therefore, in this chapter we will present a theoretical framework in which cognitive development can be analyzed as a process of learning. By learning we mean both the acquisition and structuring of knowledge. Although it is quite likely that physical maturation sets some sort of upper limit on the prospects for learning, it seems that major developmental phenomena can largely be explained in terms of learning, especially as it relates to the structuring and restructuring of knowledge. We propose that, while learning begins with the acquisition of declarative facts, it is knowledge structures which are the internal embodiment of competence. If one possesses the concept of conservation, it is because there is a knowledge structure which represents it. If one is to make sense of incoming facts, they must be interpreted by, and stored in, existing knowledge structures. When one attains some new level of competence, it is because a new knowledge structure has been formed, perhaps by combining old ones, perhaps by creating an analog of an old one, perhaps some other way.

In the first part of this chapter we briefly summarize three well-known characteristics of development which any theory must take into account. In the second section, we discuss several kinds of explanations that have often been postulated for developmental phenomena. The third section of this paper introduces theoretical memory structures and some explicit learning mechanisms which have been postulated to operate in two general theories of learning and memory. In the fourth section we speculate on how a learning theory embodying these structures and mechanisms might explain the phenomena introduced in the first section and we also discuss some related issues.

Observed Developmental Changes

We will describe some general findings from research in both the Piagetian tradition and also in the quantitative experimental tradition.

These are major phenomena that are well documented and generally accepted by developmentalists. All theories of development should start by attempting to explain one or more of these phenomena, and if a learning theory is to be successful, it must explain them as well.

Stages

Piaget and many others [*Flavell*, 1963] have observed a general and invariant sequence in development. At the highest level are the periods which represent major changes in the child's ability to represent and interact with the world. *Piaget* called them sensory-motor, preoperational, concrete operational and formal operational. Within the overall periods, *Piaget* detected a series of stages. There are six during the sensory-motor period; however, we will be concerned with the three which span the preoperational and concrete operational periods. It is during these two periods that *Piaget* noted the acquisition of the ability to utilize such concepts as classification, ordinal relations and conservation. Within a given concept, he studied a series of related tasks such as conservation of number, conservation of substance and conservation of liquid quantity.

He described the child's performance on each task as passing through three stages. During the first two stages the child tends to center on only one dimension, and only at the third stage is the ability to decenter and consider all relevant dimensions acquired. For example, in conservation of liquid, stage I children (age 4 or 5) typically base judgements of the liquid in two containers upon the height of the liquid in each container. Stage II children (age 5 or 6) often notice the discrepancy in the alternate dimension, but cannot consolidate the information provided in both dimensions and tend to vacillate between the two in their explanations. These two stages are said to be preoperational, while stage III (age 6 or 7), the successful attainment of the conservation, is said to be concrete operational. There is a systematic progression like this within each type of conservation. When children can successfully solve all such problems, they are noted to have acquired the principle of conservation.

The original data on Piagetian tasks are quite qualitative in nature. Children are described as either successful or unsuccessful at solving a particular task. Subsequent studies, using rigorous experimental manipulations, have changed and refined *Piaget's* original notions; however, the basic finding of invariant sequences has remained. For example, *Siegler* [1981] demonstrated a sequence of increasingly more accurate understandings of the balance scale and *Siegler and Robinson* [1981] did the same for conservation of number. *Scardamalia* [1977] has shown that children of a given age cannot do combinatorial problems with N dimensions, whereas they may be able to do them with (N-1) dimensions. Similar ideas were introduced by *Halford and Macdonald* [1977], who showed that young children (age 3) cannot reproduce a checkerboard pattern that requires a code length of 2, but can reproduce one that only has a code length of 1, while the complexity of the patterns which children can reproduce increases with age.

Decalage

A child may be in different stages on tasks that seemingly require the same underlying patterns of thought. For example, although children as young as 6 may be able to perform conservation of liquid tasks, they will fail on conservation of weight tasks until age 9. *Piaget* recognized this phenomenon and referred to it as horizontal decalage, but because he believed that each stage is characterized by basic underlying structures of thought which are general and not task specific, it still poses a major obstacle to his theory. The very existence of decalage makes it clear that there must be some changes in the child that allow the later forms of each concept to be acquired.

A phenomenon analagous to decalage also appears, in non-Piagetian contexts, among adults. *Newell and Simon* [1972] noted, for example, that two problems which are isomorphs (tic-tac-toe and number scrabble) can vary considerably in difficulty. In this case, the isomorphism depends upon converting the tic-tac-toe board into a magic square with all directions adding up to 15. Likewise, adults who have successfully learned how to solve the Tower of Hanoi problem will generally not be able to apply the 'principle' underlying it to another problem isomorph, such as the Tea Ceremony [*Hayes and Simon*, 1977]. Similar examples occur in conditional reasoning in adults. College students are much better at solving equivalent conditional reasoning problems when they are couched in a familiar real-world context [*Johnson-Laird and Wason*, 1970]. Such findings suggest that decalage is not a unique characteristic of the developing child and therefore that a learning mechanism underlies it.

Memory Deficits

During the last two decades, developmental psychologists, following in the footsteps of experimental psychologists, have discovered children's deficiencies in memory abilities, particularly those pertaining to short-term memory. For example, children of age 5 can usually recall only 4 digits in a digit-span task, and children of age 7 can recall about 5 digits, and so on [*Chi*, 1976]. Related to the quantitative limit in the amount of recall is a qualitative difference in the manner with which children go about memorizing items. It is typically found that children are not as apt as adults at adopting strategies to facilitate encoding and retrieval [*Kail and Hagen*, 1977]. Even when children do use a particular strategy, their pattern of rule usage is qualitatively different from that of adults. For example, instead of rehearsing items in a cumulative fashion, they do so one by one [*Ornstein and Naus*, 1978].

Explanations for Developmental Phenomena

In this section, four types of explanations for the general developmental findings we presented in the first section will be discussed. In doing so, we will present examples of theories which embody these explanations. Since most of these theories have multiple components, they will fit under more than one of the general categories we have chosen. It should be remembered, therefore, that our purpose is to highlight important notions underlying developmental theory, not to categorize the contributions of individual authors. Also, the categories themselves are not in any way mutually exclusive; they tend to overlap in many ways, and overlap with learning theory, as well. We make our own extrapolations (when possible) in instances where the authors have not explicitly tried to explain a particular type of finding.

Capacity Increase Due to Growth

The most straightforward explanation for development is that children have to reach a certain state of physical and mental maturity before they can perform a certain task. Such theories derive in general from motor development theories, such as that of *Gesell* [1928], who documented an infant's motor capabilities with increasing age. He observed that training an infant twin on a particular motor task such as stair climbing will not result in any better performance than that of the untrained twin after a given amount of growth time, such as 9 weeks [*Gesell and Thompson*, 1929]. Although young children's central nervous systems do develop in the years after birth and theories based on 'readiness from growth' are still popular in motor learning research [*Robertson*, 1978], the current trend is to move away from that notion as an explanation for intellectual development [*Gallagher and Thomas*, 1980]. Physical growth may very well set an upper limit on developmental possibilities, but it is, as *Piaget* himself noted, the child's interaction with the environment that is of crucial importance.

However, a number of theorists have proposed that a very specific and measurable increase does take place in the capacity of short-term or working memory. The forerunner of this type of theory is *Pascual-Leone* [1970], and subsequent endorsers are *Case* [1972], *Scardamalia* [1977] and *Halford and Wilson* [1980], although *Piaget* [1928] himself also recognized such limitations. The basic notion underlying this type of theory is that performance in more complex tasks requires more items to be held in short-term memory. However, the maximum size of short-term memory is quite small, no more than seven items [*Miller*, 1956], and it is difficult to see how capacity increase alone could account for more than very simple developmental changes. Thus, this idea is usually coupled with the notion that the increased capacity allows the utilization of more complex skills, and capacity increase then becomes inseparable from increases in procedural knowledge, i.e. learning. If the skills required for a task are represented as rules, for instance, the rules for more complex tasks may require more items of information in order to execute and, perhaps, more capacity for storing intermediate results. Evidence in support of such interpretations is provided by *Scardamalia* [1977] and *Halford and Macdonald* [1977], among others. However, it is quite possible for the rules themselves to be improved in ways which allow the same short-term capacity to be utilized more efficiently, and it is difficult, if not impossible, to separate these kinds of changes from actual changes in capacity. We will describe in more detail how these changes can take place in our discussion of models of memory structures and learning processes; however, an example may make this idea clearer.

Baylor and Gascon [1974] have identified at least three basic strategies representing the three stages of development in weight seriation, as shown in table I (column 1). Stage I children have a rule or rules which allow them to compare two blocks at a time. They cannot go beyond pairs, however, and so cannot seriate the blocks at all. Stage II children essentially seriate in subseries. That is, in addition to being able to compare two blocks, they have rules which can deal with groups of 3 or 4 blocks. Stage III children finally have rules that can deal with any number of blocks. The necessary goal is to find the heaviest remaining one. Since the analysis is in

Table I. Baylor and Gascon's [1974] production system analysis of weight seriation

Stage characteristics	Mean number of items in	
	conditions	actions
Stage 1: juxtaposition of couples	1.0	1.6
Stage 2: juxtaposition of subseries	1.7	1.8
Stage 3: find heaviest	1.6	1.5

the form of production rules which have several components in the condition and action side of each rule, we have calculated the mean number of components of each. As can be seen from table I (columns 2 and 3), no obvious differences can be found. Hence, at least in this analysis, the role of the capacity of working memory does not seem to apply at the level of the size of individual rules.

Decalage provides further evidence that the invariant sequences characteristic of stages are not well explained by capacity increase alone. Stage I children can consider only one dimension; stage II children are aware of both but still use only one or the other in their explanations. Thus, it might be that at stage III, they have gained the extra capacity needed to keep both dimensions in mind at one time. However, children can be at stage I or II on one task and stage III on another at the same time. For instance, conservation of liquid is attained at age 6 or 7, conservation of weight at 9 or 10, and conservation of volume at 11 or 12. Although it is quite possible to assume that differences in the actual memory demands of such tasks are responsible for decalage, it is difficult to see how the observed increases in short-term memory ability alone could account for these differences. Also, it is possible to manipulate performance abilities on these kinds of tasks. *Gelman* [1969] has shown that children younger than the expected age can perform conservation tasks if the appropriate cues are pointed out to them. These kinds of results [see *Gelman*, 1978, for others] contradict the strict notions of stages and indicate the importance of knowledge in Piagetian tasks.

The concept of increasing short-term capacity originally came, of course, from memory research and it is easier to see how capacity changes can account for memory improvements. Basically, short-term recall is seen as a direct output of the contents of working memory [*McLaughlin*, 1963].

There may be some capacity occupied by control processes but, clearly, the larger the size of short-term memory, the greater is the ability of recall. There are problems with even this seemingly simple interpretation, however. For example, the apparent short-term memory capacity of both children and adults can be manipulated by altering the nature of the stimulus materials. *Chi* [1978] has shown that children are able to recall a greater number of items than adults when the material to be recalled is familiar to them. Similarly, adults can exhibit inferior recall when the material is not familiar to them. Thus, knowledge can interact very strongly with short-term memory abilities as well.

Thus, although the capacity of short-term memory might increase, it is not possible to explain developmental differences without postulating additional changes. Specifically, these changes are changes in knowledge, both procedural skill knowledge and general factual knowledge. Whether or not there is a capacity change, the size of short-term memory is always severely limited, and one has to learn strategies to deal ever more effectively with this limitation.

Representational Changes

Another explanation often presented for developmental differences is changes in representation, changes in the way the external environment is represented in memory. The most dramatic changes are postulated in the *mode* of representation, while more continuous and gradual changes are postulated in the *availability of memory structures*. In any event, there are two basic ways these changes can take place: maturation or learning.

Changes in the Mode of Representation. Popular conceptions of this idea are those of *Piaget* [1971] and *Bruner* et al. [1966]. The most obvious representational changes are those from an enactive (or sensory-motor) mode, occurring predominantly in infancy, to imaginal, occurring predominantly in the preoperational stage, to symbolic (or linguistic), occurring between the ages of 6 and 8. There is abundant evidence to suggest that these representations are present at these ages [*Mandler*, 1981]. Our interest here, however, centers on how the changes in representational mode can explain developmental findings of stage-like transition in problem solving, decalage and quantitative improvements in memory performance. We will focus, as an example, on the shift from imaginal to symbolic representation. Since the nature of imaginal representation is assumed to be relatively static, a child at the imaginal stage cannot represent transformation, which is required in order to solve problems such as conservation. However, the existence of decalage indicates that, while a symbolic representation might be necessary, it is not sufficient to explain success on conservation and other tasks because some of them are not attained until long after this representation is well established.

How do changes from imaginal to linguistic mode account for quantitative differences in memory performance? There are several interpretations. First, the availability of the linguistic representation probably means that there are more opportunities for the modality of the stimulus material to be compatible with the mode of representation of the stored information, thus bypassing the need to continually transform the input to a mode that would be consistent with stored information. Second, the availability of another mode of representation also permits multiple encoding, thus enhancing memory due to the duplicity of storage [*Liben*, in press; *Paivio*, 1971]. Finally, perhaps the most important reason is that having linguistic representation enhances memory performance because it facilitates the use of various verbal strategies, such as rehearsal, labelling, and so on.

The mechanism that permits the representational changes to take place often is not stated explicitly. However, *Fischer* [1980] has postulated that it is the cumulative effects of small changes in memory structures. When structures reach a certain level of complexity there is a dramatic change in the kinds of information which they can interpret and represent. For instance, when sensory-motor structures become complex enough, they can represent the relationships between motor acts and their observed consequences in one structure and, thus, become imaginal. *Kosslyn* [1978] also postulates that a large number of local changes in memory structures due to interaction with the environment cause such a change. He suggests that association, comparisons, and other mental operations initially rely on imagery. However, after frequent associations and/or comparisons, they can be stored directly. So, for example, if a child is frequently asked whether a lion or a dog is bigger, then eventually the child can answer by simply storing the proposition, 'a lion is bigger than a dog', without doing an imaginal comparison. Thus, the child's knowledge base is changed through learning. According to both *Fischer's* [1980] and *Kosslyn's* [1978] notions, changes in mode of representation come about from the accumulation of specific, localized changes in memory due to frequent exposures to environmental demand, suggesting that such changes in representational preference are not unique to children but should be demonstrable in adults learning a new domain. Thus, we would interpret changes in representation not as an explanation for development, but rather as the outcome of more fundamental processes of learning and interaction with the environment.

Another reason for the inadequacy of changes in mode as an explanation for development is simply that the level of detail is far too coarse. The changes are major ones which occur at infrequent intervals. Such major changes are suitable for explaining the major periods of development; however, many of the developmental improvements take place within the framework of one representational mode. For instance, quantitative differences in memory performance continue to occur after linguistic representation becomes dominant. In addition, the premise of the theories of *Piaget* [1971] and *Bruner* et al. [1966], that an imaginal representation is primarily static, may be wrong. Data from *Marmor* [1975], *Childs and Polich* [1979], and *Kail* et al. [1980] show that children as young as 5 are capable of performing mental rotation tasks of the *Cooper and Shepard* [1973] variety. Finally, if there is a shift in the preferred representational mode, it must occur gradually, since linguistic representation is available for children as soon as they are able to use language. Thus, the shift probably reflects a gradual change in the reliance on one sort of representation over another [*Kosslyn*, 1978], suggesting that the shift is an outcome of some more fundamental processes, rather than a cause for different levels of competence. For other arguments concerning the difficulties in explaining development by a change in mode see *Carey*, [in press] and *Mandler* [in press].

Availability of New Structures. A number of theorists have proposed a gradual increase in the complexity and sophistication of memory structures, permitting a more sophisticated sort of representation that is needed for the more complex tasks [*Fischer*, 1980; *Halford and Wilson*, 1980; *Piaget*, 1972]. Change of structures has also been called a 'fundamental reorganization of conceptual framework' [*Keil*, 1981, p. 200] or changes in the 'representational format' [*Carey*, in press]. Format level changes imply that children cannot learn a concept or solve a problem until they can represent it, which must await the availability of the new higher-level structures.

Most of these theories were postulated to explain stages and decalage. That is, the level of the knowledge structure corresponds to the level of competence. *Fischer's* [1980] ideas provide a good example. He refers to the basic units of structure as sets, a concept borrowed from mathematics.

Each set controls a certain behavior or skill such as, in a very young child, grasping. More sophisticated behaviors can be built up by combining sets into larger sets. In order to acquire a conservation, such as conservation of substance, a skill set must be built up out of existing structures in successive stages. Each such set is specific to the kind of task and each new conservation must have its own set. Thus, to acquire conservation of weight requires that the child not only realize that substance is still conserved when the clay is deformed, but also attend to its weight. The ability to attend to the weights of objects can itself be a skill set, which the child may or may not already possess, but in order to solve the more advanced conservation task successfully, the child must use both sets together. The way to do this is to *intercoordinate* them, to combine them into one larger, higher-level set which now embodies the skill of conservation of weight.

Although most theorists of structural changes do not address the findings of systematic improvements in memory performance, many of them would probably propose that the limit within each level would be the source of the deficits. *Case* [1972], for example, has conducted many memory tasks which produce performance data much like those obtained in serial recall. In one task, for example, children are shown a series of N ascending numerals (such as 5, 8, 11), one at a time. They are supposed to memorize this sequence. Then, a target numeral (such as 7) is presented, and the child is asked to insert the target in its proper place in the sequence. Since the digits are not random a memory structure which can represent ascending numbers easily can improve performance, especially as it develops room for longer sequences. Indeed, with increasing age, children are able to perform this task successfully for longer sequences, indicating that structural development may take place. Thus, as *Pascual-Leone* [1970] postulated, the level of logical structures available to the child can set limits on the apparent magnitude of the working memory.

Many ideas of structural change are reasonable. There are two interrelated problems, however: (1) the vagueness with which the processes of change are described; and (2) the lack of an independently derived criterion of what constitutes a higher-level of skill, other than children's actual competence. Perhaps the notion of new and higher-level structures can be better understood when the mechanisms that induce the emergence of these levels are more clearly elucidated. Although *Fischer* [1980] describes several transition mechanisms, he describes both the structures and the transitions rather abstractly so that it is difficult to connect them to experimental findings. For instance, he allows sets to be joined in two different ways, one producing a higher-level skill and the other producing a skill at the same level. It is not clear how one determines whether a newly joined set is a higher level of skill or on the same level. *Flavell* [1972] and *Piaget* have also provided possible transition mechanisms. In general, because all of these transition mechanisms are not stated in explicit detail, it is not possible to determine whether they are unique to development or identical to learning mechanisms.

Accessibility

Another approach to explaining development is to assume that the underlying knowledge structures do not change. What changes is the child's ability to access the 'relevant' knowledge structure. *Rozin* [1976], for example, assumes that cognitive development is the increasing ability to access or apply a skill to a wider domain of tasks and situations. Accessibility actually was popularized early in the sixties when *Flavell* [1970] discussed the notion of 'mediation deficiency'. He postulated that children often realize that they need to use a specific skill (or strategy), but simply are not able to apply it to a specific task or domain. More recently, *Brown and Campione* [1981] have stressed the notion of limited accessibility in the sense that children, even when they are experts in a particular domain, can still only access this competence in that domain and not a novel one.

The notion of limited access makes a descriptive explanation of decalage quite straightforward: The child has a rule or principle, such as conservation, but must learn to access it for each individual domain, such as liquid quantity. The same explanation can be given for children's inability to generalize strategies learned in memory tasks, and for the exceptional, but domain-specific, memory performance of expert children [*Chi*, 1978]. However, simply labelling a phenomenon does not really explain it. The concept of access simply raises further difficult questions. Is accessing knowledge structures a cognitive ability which is separate from these structures? If so, we need to know what form this ability takes and how it changes. For instance, why does the ability to access conservation take a particular sequence? An alternative explanation, which eliminates the need for a separate cognitive function, is that the observed phenomena are a consequence of the knowledge structures themselves. The following example illustrates the point.

Lawler [1981], while observing his daughter's development, documented a phenomenon which can easily be called lack of access, although he did not explicitly use that term. His daughter learned to do mental calculation involving money. At the same time, she also learned to do mental arithmetic involving pure numbers by breaking them into multiples of ten and counting up the remainders. She did not, however, connect the two techniques. For example, when asked to add 75 and 26, she said 'seventy, ninety, ninety-six, ninety-seven,...' [p. 4] and continued counting to one-hundred-one. When the question was posed in terms of money, however, she said 'That's three quarters, four, and a penny, a dollar one' [p. 4]. *Lawler* [1981] refers to these separate skills as microworlds. In both cases, she completed the sums by counting the leftover units. Thus, she had two distinct microworlds, with different conditions for their activation to accomplish what might seem to be the same logical task, and which apparently accessed the same counting skill to complete their actions. Only later did *Lawler* [1981] observe moments of insight when his daughter first noticed that she could combine her tens microworld with her money microworld.

Here we see skills that might seem to an adult to be part of the same skill, but which are actually separate. Access to the money microworld is limited to situations where money is explicitly mentioned. However, there is no need to postulate that there is some general access mechanism which causes this phenomenon. Rather it is the structure of the microworlds themselves and wider access is gained by a structural change, combining the two microworlds in some way. Thus, although lack of access is certainly a real phenomenon, it can be seen to be only a description of the effects of changing knowledge structures. Later, we will discuss several mechanisms by which knowledge structures might change through learning. One of them, *generalization*, has particular relevance to accessibility because it widens the range of application of rules. Here again, however, wider access is the result of a change in knowledge structure.

Knowledge Differences

A factor which must surely be considered in development is the simple accumulation of knowledge; older children clearly know more than younger ones [*Chi*, 1976] and, just as clearly, they obtain this knowledge through learning. Some have tried to make a distinction between theories of knowledge acquisition and theories involving structural change, labeling the former quantitative and the latter qualitative. Thus, whether the representation is a network organized into schemas [*Chi*, in press, a; *Chi and Koeske*, 1983], events [*Nelson*, 1978], scripts [*Mandler*, in press; *Nelson*, et al. this volume], production rules [*Newell*, 1973] or some other form, if new knowledge is simply added to the existing structure, the result is only a quantitative change. However, this view is probably too naive. For instance, in a rule-based representation, new knowledge means new rules and, even though they are in the same representation, they can clearly produce a qualitative change in the overall system [*Young*, 1978]. Indeed, simply adding to any structure can make it more powerful and produce an apparent qualitative change. Thus, while the qualitative-quantitative distinction is useful for our purpose of highlighting developmental explanations, it should not be taken too literally. There are two subcategories of knowledge difference theories to be discussed below.

Rule Adoption and Strategy Usage. One type of knowledge in which differences are found is procedural knowledge, knowledge of how to do things, which can be represented as rules. The changes in children's performance at different ages are explained in terms of different rules that they use at different stages. Some of the most explicit and detailed descriptions of rule use were presented by *Baylor and Gascon* [1974] on weight seriation, *Klahr and Wallace* [1972] on class inclusion and *Young* [1978] on length seriation. Essentially, each of these theories is a simulation (whether implemented on the computer or not) of the task performance, using different rules (or sets of processes) for a different level of cognitive attainment. What the simulation accomplishes is to describe the rules used by children at each stage of competence and to verify that they will indeed produce the observed behavior. We have already described *Baylor and Gascon's* [1974] analysis of the rules in table I. A similar line of reasoning is the rule assessment method of *Siegler* [1976, 1981]. Using this technique, *Siegler* was able to assess the precise rules children were using by the particular pattern of correct and erroneous responses they gave in a particular task, such as the balance scale [*Siegler,* 1981] and conservation of number [*Siegler and Robinson,* 1981].

Usage of a particular strategy or set of rules is also a common and prevalent explanation for memory improvements with age. A strategy here is usually defined as a set of processes, like rehearsal, that has been shown in the adult literature to be beneficial to remembering. And development has been shown to exhibit progressive improvement in the use of such strategies. There is an abundance of evidence and review articles on the topic [*Kail and Hagen,* 1977; *Ornstein,* 1978]. The difference between the notions here and those used in the Piagetian research is that, in the former case, we are talking about the adoption and elaboration of a particular set of rules (such as rehearsal) with increasing age, whereas in the latter case, we are talking about the adoption and use of new and more sophisticated rules at each stage of development.

Methods of assessing rule usage are very important in developmental research. At the very least, this approach allows the researcher to adequately describe in great detail the types of rules or strategies a child at a particular level is using. The intention of the rule usage approach has been to identify which components of the rules change. The implicit assumption is that once the rules of different levels are described, one can compare them to see where the differences lie and thereby understand how one rule can be transformed into another. However, transition mechanisms and transformation rules have simply not been forthcoming from this line of research. For example, it is not clear how *Baylor and Gascon's* [1974] weight seriation rules can be transformed from stage to stage, what kind of learning rules are needed, and so on. On the other hand, *Siegler's* [1981] balance scale rules do build upon each other as do *Siegler and Robinson's* [1981] number conservation rules. Thus, it may be that, at times, fairly direct learning processes act to produce modified versions of existing rules, while at other times, entirely new rules are created through the mediation of other changes in knowledge structures.

General World Knowledge. The other subcategory of knowledge which changes during development is factual, declarative knowledge of the world; clearly, children's world knowledge is less elaborated than adults'. Consequently, this gap must somehow affect children's performance in a variety of tasks. This kind of reasoning has been applied to both experimental memory tasks and Piagetian results.

Many theories have recognized the importance of world knowledge in a general way [*Brown,* 1975; *Olson,* 1973]. Some are more explicit and explain the consequences of the lack of general world knowledge in terms of chunk sizes [*Chi,* 1976; *Dempster,* 1978; *Simon,* 1972] and possibly slower access [*Chi,* 1976]. However, it was not until knowledge was explicitly manipulated that the factor of general knowledge came into prominence in developmental research [*Chi,* 1978; *Lindberg,* 1980]. Because it is difficult to define what exactly constitutes general world knowledge, experimental investigations have focused on knowledge in specific domains. Depending on how much initial knowledge the child is equipped with, researchers are able to reverse developmental trends, and/or eliminate robust developmental incapacities [*Chi,* in press, b; *Gelman,* 1978]. The importance of this knowledge component is becoming more and more convincing as greater numbers of isomorphs are appearing between the performance of a child compared to the adult versus the performance of the adult novice compared to the adult expert [*Brown,* 1982; *Chi,* in press, a].

The effect of inadequate declarative knowledge on Piagetian tasks has also been suggested by *Siegler* [1976], and more recently by *Carey* [in press], who used the same logic to postulate explanations for a variety of tasks, such as class inclusion and hypothesis testing and generation. Clearly, the child must possess some factual knowledge about the components of a task before mastering it. There is undoubtedly some effect of factual knowledge involved in decalage as well. For instance, a child who does not know what volume is will undoubtedly have great trouble mastering its conservation.

Memory Structures and Learning Mechanisms

In this section we will describe some theoretical memory structures, specifically, node-link networks, production rules and schemas. These structures have been used in a number of different theories and explanations, but we will be concerned with two which have been implemented, at least partially, on computers: ACT by *Anderson* [1976] and ASN (active structural network) by *Norman and Rumelhart* [1975]. We are interested in these two because they contain explicit learning processes to acquire, structure and restructure knowledge and because these processes have, at least to some extent, been tested and shown to be successful.

Memory Structures

Networks. Networks of nodes and links (often called propositional networks) have been very popular because they capture the associative nature of memory very effectively [*Anderson,* 1976; *Anderson and Bower,* 1973; *Collins and Loftus,* 1975; *Collins and Quillian,* 1969; *Norman and Rumelhart,* 1975; *Rumelhart* et al. 1972; *Quillian,* 1966]. Each node stands for a particular concept and the links stand for the associations or relations between nodes. Learning is the insertion of new nodes into their proper places and the acquisition of new links between existing nodes. In some models, the links can have strengths which represent the strength of association between concepts. In this case, learning can also be the strengthening of links. Alternatively, increasing strength of association might be represented by establishing multiple links between nodes [*Chi and Koeske,* 1983]. Networks are very natural representations for factual, declarative knowledge, but they can also be used to represent procedural knowledge, as we will explain in more detail shortly.

Production Rules. Production rules [*Klahr and Wallace,* 1972; *Newell,* 1973; *Newell and Simon,* 1972] can be thought of as generalized stimulus-response pairs [*Anderson,* 1976]. Each one consists of a condition side and an action side and they are often informally represented as *if=then* pairs. *If* the condition side matches the contents of short-term memory *then* the action is taken. The condition side can contain constants, which must match specific items, or variables, which can match general classes of items. The actions are generally modifications to memory. This match-action structure makes production rules ideal for representing procedural knowledge. Items can be rehearsed in short-term memory, moved from long-term to short-term memory or moved from short-term to long-term, i.e. memorized. Also goals and subgoals can be set. Since production systems are usually used for modelling cognitive activities, the processes of getting stimuli into short-term memory and controlling overt physical actions are usually ignored. In principle, however, there is no reason why they could not be modelled as well [*Klahr and Wallace,* 1972].

Production systems have several characteristics which make them quite useful for modelling human behavior and learning. First, they explicitly take the contents of short-term memory into account. This means they can handle attentional processes quite naturally. Also, because it is the contents of this memory that are generally 'seen' by such techniques as protocol analysis [*Ericsson and Simon,* 1980], comparing models with experimental data may be facillitated.

Second, they can behave very flexibly. This occurs mainly because the order of application of the rules depends upon the contents of short-term memory; one rule does not explicitly call another rule. It is only through changing the contents of this memory and setting goals that rules affect the flow of control. This style of control means that a production system can be easily interruptable. For instance, if an important piece of data enters short-term memory from the environment while some behavior is ongoing, an entirely unrelated production can match, initiating behavior appropriate to the new situation. This rapid, direct response to incoming stimuli is often referred to as stimulus-driven or bottom-up processing. Similarly, a series of productions with similar but not identical conditions can exist so that subtle differences in situations, which result in small differences in short-term memory, can cause variations in behavior. Thus, a production system can respond very quickly to important changes in a situation and very flexibly to small differences in familiar situations.

Third, production systems, although they are flexible and interruptible due to incoming data, can maintain a focus of attention and ignore irrelevant stimuli once a particular behavior is initiated. This is because, in most systems, at least one element of each condition is a goal and groups of productions which are related have the same goal. Goals and subgoals, as well as other elements, placed in short-term memory by the actions of productions strongly constrain which conditions can match. This style of processing is referred to as concept-driven or top-down. Just as it is necessary to respond to important stimuli, it is necessary to ignore unimportant inputs and maintain a focus of attention. There is abundant evidence that human behavior results from a combination of bottom-up and top-down processing, and it is very important for any model to be able to capture both at the same time.

The fourth useful characteristic of production systems is that it is relatively easy to add new rules to a system without radically altering its behavior. One reason for this characteristic is that each rule must contain a relatively small piece of knowledge. The condition side can never exceed the capacity of short-term memory, and the action side, since it usually operates on this memory as well, is constrained to be of similar size. Another reason is that rules never call each other directly, so there is no need to change other rules to call the new one or decide which rules the new one should call. Also, in many production systems, the matching process is conceived to be a parallel one in which all condition sides are tested at once, so there is no need to place a new rule in a particular location relative to the other rules. If it matches, it will be found wherever it is. The obvious importance of the ability to add new rules easily is that learning can be modelled in this way. Each new rule is a small incremental change and it is the accumulation of a lot of new rules over time that causes significant changes in the behavior of the system. In fact, new rules can be added through the action of other rules in the system [*Waterman,* 1975] so that production systems can actually learn.

Schemas. Basically, a schema is an organized unit or structure of memory that contains some body of related knowledge. Quite some time ago *Bartlett* [1932] used the schema concept to explain recall for stories.

However, most of the work on schemas and related structures, such as scripts [*Nelson* et al., this volume] and frames, is relatively recent [*Anderson* et al., 1981; *Minsky,* 1975; *Rosch and Lloyd,* 1978; *Rumelhart and Norman,* 1976; *Rumelhart and Ortony,* 1977; *Schank and Abelson,* 1977]. There is a wide variety of possible implementations of this general idea; however, only a few characteristics of schemas are important for our purposes. Schemas have slots or variables into which incoming data can fit. If enough slots are filled in a particular schema, it becomes active. As with production rules, this is often referred to as stimulus-driven or bottom-up processing. Once a schema is active, it can cause top-down processing of incoming information. Unfilled slots guide attention to relevant data, while factual information present in the schema can fill in gaps or even override inconsistent data. Although it is not necessary to specify how an individual schema is organized in order to understand how they work, it is important to note that schemas can be hierarchically organized. Two or more related schemas can be joined together into one higher level schema, and an existing schema, as it becomes more complex through learning, might develop subschemas.

To illustrate how schemas might operate, consider a child learning about a new dinosaur from a picture card. If the picture were mixed in with a group of other kinds of animals, visual features of the animal would have to fit into slots in the dinosaur schema in order to activate it; the child would have to recognize it as a dinosaur. On the other hand, if he or she knows initially what the general subject is, the dinosaur schema is already activated. In that case, the slots in this schema guide attention to various features of the picture which previous experience and learning have shown to be important. Thus, the child may look to see if it walks on two or four feet, if it has lots of sharp teeth or not, if it has a long or short neck, if it has some kind of armor and so on. Once the schema is filled in with this information, a copy of it (perhaps only partial) can be placed in long-term memory to create a specific trace of the dinosaur and its characteristics.

If the child has learned enough to discriminate different categories of dinosaurs, the overall schema may contain a set of subschemas which represent them. Thus, an upright dinosaur with a short neck and sharp teeth could fit the ferocious meat-eater schema, allowing the child to infer that it is in fact a meat-eater. This inference will enable the newly learned dinosaur to be linked with other examples from the same subschema. When a schema is active, if a piece of information (such as whether it has sharp teeth) is not provided, then facts stored in the schema can be used. Thus, if the teeth are not visible, but enough other information is present to activate the meat-eater schema, sharp teeth will be inferred. This is generally referred to as a default value.

Because schemas organize units of knowledge, they are at a higher conceptual level than production rules or networks. This level is a very useful one for many purposes because the explicit specification of individual pieces of knowledge and their interrelationships is difficult, in many cases impossible and, in many cases, such detail is simply not necessary. If a detailed specification of the structure and contents of schemas is needed, they can be implemented using either production rules or a network or a combination of both. For instance, a set of nodes in a network that is very tightly interrelated via multiple links [*Chi and Koeske,* 1983] can be a schema. Also, a group of production rules with the same goal element can be viewed as a schema, with the variables in the conditions of the rules representing the slots. The next two sections give some more examples of how schemas have been implemented.

Processes of Learning in ACT

The ACT system [*Anderson,* 1976] is designed to provide an explicit division between procedural and declarative knowledge. For this reason, it contains both production rules to represent procedures and a node-link network to represent factual knowledge. As in many network models, only part of the network is accessible, active, at any one time. A small area which is the most active represents short-term memory and is what is accessed by the condition sides of the rules. The activation spreads via the links over time in order to capture the free-associative nature of memory, and one type of learning is the strengthening of links which allows activation to flow more readily.

Although ACT is not explicitly a schema model, it is possible to build schemas into it in various ways. For instance, *Anderson* et al. [1981] give two examples of possible kinds. The first is a declarative schema which is simply an area of the network containing an organized body of factual knowledge. In fact, it is difficult to imagine how a network of knowledge could exist without identifiable schemas of this type. In this case, general production rules can access and use the schemas. Depending upon the current contents of short-term memory, the same productions can access different schemas, and the same schema can be used in different ways by different rules, to solve a problem by working forward or backward, for instance. We should note that this organization is the one we currently prefer in our own modelling attempts [*Chi and Koeske,* 1983]. The second type of schema makes the connection between declarative and procedural knowledge more explicit. In this case, each schema has its own *schematizing productions* associated with it. The purpose of these productions is to determine if incoming stimuli fit into the slots and, if so, to activate the schema. Thus, while schemas might be modelled using the variables of production rule conditions as slots, the slots in this model are nodes with which the productions link the appropriate incoming stimuli. Once a particular schema is active, its *procedural attachments* specify procedures which can act on the items in the slots. These attachments are themselves specified very much like the main schema and might be thought of as subschemas. They specify the actual set of production rules to be used to carry out the procedure.

Acquisition of Declarative Knowledge. The accumulation of declarative knowledge must be assumed to be a fundamental learning process available to humans of all ages. Indeed, *Anderson* [1981] makes a strong case that this must be the first stage of all learning. Hence, production rules should exist which enable the system to store new declarative knowledge in the network. *Neves and Anderson* [1981] refer to this process as *declarative encoding.* Modification of the declarative knowledge, once it exists, can be accomplished in ACT by production rules which explicitly change certain structures. In fact, as we pointed out earlier, many actions of the productions constitute modifications of the declarative knowledge structure.

Acquisition of Procedural Knowledge. In ACT, procedural knowledge is acquired, after practice, through the conversion of declarative knowledge. *Anderson* [1981] refers to this transformation as *knowledge compilation* which consists of two components: *proceduralization* and *composition.* It begins with the specific knowledge necessary to perform a skill in declarative form in memory (or perhaps still in an external medium such as a textbook). General interpretive productions, productions which contain mostly general variables in their conditions, must be used to access the declarative knowledge. For example, suppose a student is learning geometry. He or she may know declaratively that in order to prove two triangles congruent, the side-angle-side (SAS) postulate is useful. This might simply be an isolated fact represented by some nodes and links or, if the student is a little further along, it might be a part of the declarative schema for SAS.

When such a problem is presented, there is, in active memory, along with various features of the problem, the very general goal of finding a way to solve it. In order to proceed, interpretive productions must find in declarative memory knowledge which has associated with it the information that it can achieve this goal. When this step is complete, the problem solver has in active memory the goal to apply the SAS postulate. Again, general productions must search declarative memory to find information, this time about how to apply SAS. This cycle continues until the problem is solved. It is very slow and halting because information must be searched out, brought into and kept in active memory at every step of the way. At times, active memory must be rehearsed to keep important information from decaying before it can be used and, at other times, the solution path attempted may overload active memory and cause important information to be lost. In addition, because very general productions are being used, they may at times retrieve declarative knowledge which seems to be useful but which, in fact, leads down blind alleys, necessitating backtracking.

Once the student has had some practice using the SAS postulate, copies of the general interpretive productions can be created with specific knowledge of the SAS postulate embedded in them. Essentially, this *proceduralization* is done by replacing variables (in both the condition and action sides) with the items from declarative memory to which they have been matching. For instance, the student might attain a new production which says: *if* you want to prove two triangles congruent, *then* try SAS. One cycle of searching declarative memory and bringing items into short-term memory is thereby eliminated, making the process faster and more reliable.

Production rules which already exist in memory can be modified by *composition*. Productions which have been applying in the same sequence whenever a skill is performed are collapsed into fewer, more powerful ones, essentially by concatenating conditions and actions of the individual rules. The productions involved might be the general interpretive productions as well as the proceduralized productions. Composition obviously results from practice, and it manifests the properties inherent in practice. First, once productions are concatenated, fewer are now needed to accomplish the same thing. Thus, the process happens faster and there is less chance of a 'wrong' rule getting into the sequence. Also, since fewer accesses of working memory are needed, there is less chance of forgetting elements and there is more short-term memory capacity available, allowing other features of the situation to be noticed which might lead to further improvements. In sum, the skill becomes faster and more reliable, which is the result when one practices. The overall result of these two processes might be to create a single production rule which automatically causes the proper correspondences between sides and angles to be made whenever a triangle congruence problem is encountered.

Further practice continues to improve performance through the general process of *tuning*. *Generalization* and *specialization* can cause more accurate versions of productions to be created and further composition can also occur. To generalize, the range of items which will match the conditions is increased, such as by replacing constants with variables. For example, suppose that a child has the following production:

'*If* the goal is to remember, and there is a string of digits, *then* repeat them one by one'.

Generalization can occur by replacing the condition 'a string of digits' by the variable 'a string of items'. Specialization works in reverse; general variables are replaced with more specific items. The net result of all of these processes for our geometry student might be to create a rule whose condition side is specific to just those triangle congruence problems with features suitable for SAS. Thus, the student may be able to recognize how to do such problems without any apparent conscious effort.

Processes of Learning in ASN

Unlike ACT, ASN uses only a node-link network to represent all knowledge. This network is organized into schemas with the characteristics we noted earlier, slots and a hierarchical structure. *Rumelhart and Norman* [1976] propose that these schemas allow one to organize, expand, understand and store inputs, as in our dinosaur example. Similarly they allow one to interpret memories when they are recalled. They also can control actions [*Rumelhart and Norman*, 1982].

The unitary representation allows the same knowledge to be both procedural and declarative at the same time. Thus, a dinosaur schema may consist of the node 'dinosaur' linked to the node 'ferocious meat-eater', with links from this node to 'upright', 'lots of sharp teeth' and 'short neck'. This structure, which is probably part of a more general dinosaur schema, could be accessed as declarative knowledge. On the other hand, this same structure can represent a set of instructions for determining if a dinosaur is a ferocious meat-eater. ASN contains a general interpreter which can trace through a set of links like this and cause the general actions of checking the teeth, and so on, to take place.

Rumelhart and Norman [1976] have proposed two general types of learning based upon schemas. Like *Anderson*, they believe acquisition of declarative facts comes first. They call it *accretion*. Existing schemas are used to store items in their proper places in the network. The other type of learning consists of several processes which operate at the schema level. A *tuning* process fairly similar to that in ACT can occur. *Generalization* here occurs within a schema by increasing the range of items which will fit slots, and *specialization* happens by decreasing their range or by replacing them with specific default values.

Schemas can also produce new schemas, a process *Rumelhart and Norman* [1976] call *restructuring*. This can be accomplished in two ways. *Patterned generation* is the creation of a new schema by modifying an old one. Thus, if no existing schemas fit a given situation well enough, a new one is created using the one that fits the best. This process can be viewed as learning by analogy [*Rumelhart and Norman*, 1981]. *Schema induction* is the creation of a new schema from two or more older ones which tend to occur together. This process is characterized as a sort of 'aha' phenomenon involving insight, and presumably occurs rarely.

Summary of Learning Mechanisms

There are many similarities in the learning mechanisms proposed for these two models. An accumulation of declarative knowledge occurs in both, as well as complex learning involving refining and restructuring of knowledge. Existing knowledge can be tuned, either through specialization or generalization, and new structures can be built from old, either through generation of analogous structures, or through the combination and concatenation of old ones. This particular set of mechanisms of learning is not novel. *Flavell* [1972] described many of these ideas, and so did *Gagné* [1968], and more recently *Fischer* [1980]. The uniqueness of the two models that we have discussed derives from the specificity with which their mechanisms are described. Our hypothesis for the time being is that either one of these models is perfectly adequate to simulate development. In fact, it may well be useful to combine ideas from both of them. Schemas are very useful for describing general units of behavior, like the sets in *Fischer's* [1980] theory, and they can, in turn, be described as groups of production rules when a more specific analysis of structure is needed.

Interpretations from a Learning Framework

One of the difficulties in modelling development or any other important psychological change, such as the acquisition of expertise, is that there is an incredible amount of experience and knowledge involved in the change. Thus, a true developmental learning model, one which has the ability to acquire adult intelligence, is improbable if not impossible. However, if the same small set of processes is at work regardless of the domain or stage of development, a basic understanding is possible. *Keil* [1981] has pointed out that some set of cognitive constraints, constraints inherent in learning processes rather than in the knowledge to be learned, seems to be necessary in order to explain the efficiency with which we learn. How would children learn rules for generating language, for instance, if any possible generalization of what they hear is equally possible? Perhaps a small set of learning processes, such as those we have described, operating on a basic set of knowledge structures, provides these constraints. These processes will build up structures which are immensely complex, but which are based on a few principles.

If this is true, then models of limited domains and limited changes can illuminate the wider course of development. Smaller domains of increasing competence have been modelled successfully by changes in the knowledge structures available to the child. We have previously mentioned the success of the rule assessment method [*Siegler*, 1981], for instance. As another example, *Riley* et al. [in press] have modelled the knowledge required to perform various kinds of simple algebra word problems. They identified schemas which guide the representation of three basic problem types: change, compare and combine. *Riley* et al. [in press] were able to explain the performance of each child by showing that older children tend to have more accurate and complete versions of each schema. Although their model and the rule assessment models cannot explain how these different conceptual structures are acquired, it is clear that the components of the learning mechanisms proposed in the ASN and ACT models can eventually accommodate these transitions. With these thoughts in mind, we can now consider how a learning theory can explain the phenomena we described in the first section, as well as some others.

Stages and Decalage

One interesting consequence of a general learning model is that stages and decalage are really manifestations of a few underlying assumptions, but at different levels. In general, we assume: (1) only a small amount of new knowledge can be learned at any one time; (2) this new knowledge must be interpreted by and stored in existing knowledge structures; (3) new structures, when they are needed, are created from old ones, and (4) knowledge tends to be specific to the context in which it was learned.

Thus, when a child is learning a new skill, certain prerequisite knowledge and knowledge structures must already exist. If they do not, they must be learned first. For instance, *Siegler* [1981] showed that for a child to progress from a balance scale rule involving only weight to one involving distance as well, it is necessary for the child to learn to encode distance first, before using it in a rule. This idea was essentially proposed by *Gagné* [1968]. Specifically, he theorized that learning is necessarily hierarchical in nature; that in order to learn a concept such as conservation of liquid, a series of component pieces of knowledge must be learned first. These components may be procedural rules or declarative concepts, and each one, in turn, requires the existence of other subsidiary pieces of knowledge. For example, in order for conservation of liquid to be mastered, he proposed that a rule stating that the volume of liquid is determined jointly by its length, width and height (in a rectangular container) is necessary. He further proposed that a necessary preliminary to learning this rule is to learn three rules stating that if one dimension is held constant, changing one other dimension results in a compensatory change in the remaining one. The actual rules he proposed may not be correct; however, his proposal shows graphically how the content of the knowledge itself and the limits on how much can be learned at any one time create a stage-like learning sequence. This view is rather similar to *Fischer's* [1980] notion of *intercoordination* of sets and *Rumelhart and Norman's* [1976] *schema induction* in which a new schema is created from two or more older ones, as well as to *Flavell's* [1972] *hierarchical integration*. It can also be related to *composition* in *Anderson's* [1981] terms. The component rules would be learned individually and used separately at first, until, with practice they were 'added up' to form the conservation rule. Thus, stages may result from the interaction of constraints inherent in the knowledge being learned and in how knowledge is acquired and structured.

To understand decalage, it is necessary to assume that when conservation of X is learned, what is learned is a knowledge structure specific to X, not a general concept. That is not to say that there might not be a general concept of conservation which can be learned; however, such a concept is very complex due to the number of things which are conserved and the number of transformations under which they are conserved. Some decalage may result because each new task really requires a more complex knowledge structure. For instance, conservation of weight can not be mastered if conservation of substance has not already been mastered, and the weight structure may be built up from the substance structure. Other kinds of decalage may result because subsidiary knowledge can not be mastered. Conservation of volume is typically not mastered until age 10 or 11, and it obviously cannot be mastered if the concept of volume itself is not understood. A study of volume alone might well show a sequence of preliminary knowledge states, taking some years to master, very similar to other sequences which have been noted.

Since learning is a process shared by adults, phenomena analogous to stages and decalage should be observable at all ages. We have already noted that there are observations in the adult literature which are analogous to decalage, such as lack of transfer on problem isomorphs. Since we see stages as simply a necessary step-by-step learning process, they too are evident in adults. An adult can no more learn a piece of knowledge without its prerequisites than can a child. However, an adult knowledge base is far more elaborate, and the kinds of new concepts and skills adults acquire are more complex than the simple sort of tasks *Piaget* pioneered. Thus, pinpointing the knowledge required to learn an adult skill is far more difficult and so is determining whether an adult has some or all of that knowledge. Also, for a more complex skill, there are undoubtedly many more possible sequences of knowledge states leading to the same result, making determination of the existence of any such sequences all the more difficult. In fact, a number of authors have pointed out that multiple pathways are probably available to developing children as well [*Fischer*, 1980; *Longeot*, cited in *Vuyk*, 1981]. Thus, when considering the invariant sequences thought to be characteristic of development it is important to remember that the invariance may be on a more abstract level than that of the actual chain of knowledge states. The constraints inherent in knowledge and the characteristics of learning may only limit development to a series of possible sequences, not a single invariant one.

Levels of Understanding

An interesting finding, related to stages and decalage, is that of levels of understanding. *Piaget* noted that once a child has acquired a particular principle, a rapid broadening of understanding of related phenomena takes place. As *Fischer* [1980, p. 485] put it, 'As a child moves into a new level, he or she will show rapid change, but once the level has been attained, he or she will show slower change'. There are a number of factors which can be seen from a learning perspective to produce this sort of effect. Although we have noted that knowledge is specific to the context in which it is learned, that is not to say that it is absolutely specific. When a child learns conservation of substance, for instance, it is unlikely that what is learned is a piece of knowledge that relates only to a specific piece of clay deformed in a certain way by a certain person, etc. Although this knowledge is not so general that it represents an abstract understanding of 'conservation', it must have some generality or it would never apply after the first time it was learned. The schema slot or production rule condition element which matches the deformed substance, for instance, should at least cover all kinds of clay and probably more substances that are similar to clay. By the same token, there are many elements of the situation, such as the time of day and the particular location, which should not be incorporated into the knowledge structure at all. How all this happens is not clear; however, there is evidence that children naturally tend to generalize their experiences [*Nelson* et al., this volume]. At any rate, newly acquired skills and knowledge are automatically ready to be used in situations which are somehow similar to the one in which they were learned, thus, a rapid broadening of understanding can proceed from the acquisition of one new structure.

The phenomenon of rapid change can also occur when new structures are created from old ones. For instance, in ACT, if two productions are found to be potentially applicable in a certain situation and they have enough in common in terms of the structures of their conditions and actions, a new *generalization* of the two can be produced. Of course, if this new production captured only what was in the previous two and nothing more, it would produce identical behavior. This is not the case, however, because specific elements in the two productions are converted to more general ones in the new production. Two different constants might be replaced by a variable; two different variables might be replaced by a more general variable. Thus, the new production has a wider applicability than the two on which it is based, and although it may well need to be refined through *discrimination* to finally achieve the proper scope, it has the potential for allowing wider understanding. Schemas can also be generalized by widening the scope of individual slots. In addition, new schemas, based on old ones, can be created through *patterned generation*. When no schema can be found which successfully applies to a given situation, a new one is created based upon one that partially fits. It is important, of course, that a schema exists which does partially fit. Another way of saying this is that the new situation is analogous to a familiar one.

Hence, once a new structure is formed, it allows a new level of understanding into many related problems. This happens both because the new structure itself has some generality built in and because a given structure can spawn many new related ones through various processes, which might be summed up as learning by analogy. At first, there is a relatively large area of related problems and situations to which the new structure or analogous ones can apply and there is a rapid burst of new understanding; however, as the area remaining is quickly reduced, the process slows down.

Although we propose that new levels of understanding result from learning, we should emphasize that this does not mean that they cannot appear abruptly. It may require months or years to accumulate enough new facts and subsidiary structures to allow the creation of an important new structure, but once all of that is available, the proper situational demands can cause it to be built very rapidly. For instance, *Norman* [1978] has proposed that sudden insight, the 'aha' phenomenon, occurs due to *restructuring* of existing knowledge. He points out that there need be no addition of knowledge at all during this process and it might occur due to the demands of a particular situation, as in a Socratic tutorial. A similar process seems to take place in the development of knowledge in general, such as scientific knowledge. For instance, it took 100 years from the time that the Academy of Experiments in Florence discovered that freezing and boiling take place instantaneously at a certain 'degree of heat' until *Black* was able to differentiate heat from temperature [*Carey*, in press]. During this time, the discovery of many facts about heat and temperature set the stage for *Black's* realization.

Memory Deficits

There are two basic ways in which learning can affect memory performance: the acquisition of memory strategies and the acquisition of new knowledge per se. There is considerable evidence that both of these effects are important. In the case of strategies, the most commonly used example is rehearsal of items in short-term memory. Young children may not use it at all, while somewhat older ones may use it idiosyncratically or only in certain situations. Numerous efforts have been made to teach rehearsal and, indeed, it can be taught, although a common finding is that subjects will still not use it spontaneously. The important point, however, is that this strategy and, no doubt others, can be learned and will improve memory performance. There is evidence that failure to use it spontaneously may be the result of the unavailability of necessary content knowledge [*Chi*, in press, a].

The effect of content knowledge on memory has already been noted. We have shown that it is possible to reverse adult and child memory performance if the material to be recalled is familiar to the child and unfamiliar to the adult [*Chi*, 1978]. As an extreme example, consider the task of remembering a series of words containing one which is completely unfamiliar. In the case of this word, only its constituent sounds are familiar. Thus, while the other words might each activate one node representing the internal concept for which that word stands, the unfamiliar one activates a series of nodes representing its constituent sounds, thereby occupying several slots in short-term memory. More generally, the more familiar material is, the greater is the number of links between concept nodes and the more likely it is that several items can be grouped under one node. Each group of items can be called a declarative schema or a chunk [*Simon*, 1974]. *Chase and Simon* [1973a, b], for instance, found that chess masters can remember fairly complicated chess positions very accurately with only a 5-second exposure because they group the pieces into a few chunks. Only the nodes representing the chunks need to be in short-term memory and when the individual pieces are to be recalled, each chunk can be retrieved from long-term memory and unpacked. In addition, the greater number of links to a node resulting from greater familiarity might simply make access to that node easier and faster [*Chi*, 1976], so that more items can be rehearsed or retrieved in the same amount of time. Thus, the contents and structure of declarative memory have a very strong impact on short-term memory ability.

An outstanding example of the effects of both knowledge and strategies on memory skills is *Chase and Ericsson's* [1981] subject S.F. He was able to learn, through heroic amounts of practice, to recall as many as about 80 random digits, presented verbally at one per second. *Chase and Ericsson* [1981] have shown convincingly that his performance was due to three basic components: (1) a large store of factual knowledge related to numbers, (2) a retrieval structure in long-term memory, and (3) very highly refined encoding and retrieval strategies. The factual knowledge base he used was basically an extensive knowledge of times for various track events of different lenghts. He used 11 different distances from half-mile to marathon and several categories of times for each, such as world records and his own bests. He developed a highly skillful procedure to group the incoming digits and relate them to this knowledge base. For instance, 356 might be encoded as his old coach's best time for the mile (3:56).

This idea is not as simple as it may seem, however, because of the rapid sequential presentation of the digits. At first, he had to collect a series of digits and decide how to group them and what kind of running time to relate them to. Such conscious decisions require short-term memory space and take time to complete and, so, interfere with subsequent digits. As time progressed, he developed a highly automatic discrimination procedure which operated on each digit as it came in, successively narrowing down the number of possibilities. He also developed a retrieval structure, which *Chase and Ericsson* [1981] characterize as a directly addressable hierarchical long-term memory structure, rather like a schema. It specified how the digits were to be grouped before presentation began, eliminating any need for concurrent grouping decisions, provided a structure into which the numbers could be stored directly without having to use short-term memory and provided the means for ordering the groups upon retrieval. Thus, each group of digits was linked to a semantic structure representing the running-time mnemonic as well as to the retrieval structure through the use of highly specialized and efficient memory procedures. Not only did this structure enable SF to recall as many as 80 digits in one trial, he was also able to recall nearly all of the digit groups from an entire 1-hour session by accessing them through his 11 running-time categories. Although this is a highly specialized example, it indicates very clearly how important knowledge, knowledge structures and procedural skills are in simple memory tasks, such as a span task.

Learning to Learn

The importance of the products of learning in memorization skills brings up a broader question: Are there fundamental invariant learning processes or can these processes themeselves undergo changes? Although, S.F. 'learned to learn' strings of digits, there is no reason to believe that his more fundamental processes, such as generalization and discrimination, underwent any changes. However, in systems such as ACT and ASN, since the learning processes themselves can be represented as rules or schemas, they can thereby be accessible to each other. Thus, as *Langley and Simon* [1981] point out, a discrimination rule might act upon a generalization rule to produce a new rule which makes more accurate generalizations, perhaps because it is specific to a particular domain. A large supply of new versions of learning rules could be created which would be better suited to current learning demands upon the developing child or adult and which would make learning faster and more efficient.

This proposal is clearly speculative and such changes may be nearly impossible to detect and/or unnecessary because changes in strategies and knowledge can have a profound impact on learning. Note that we are making a distinction between basic learning processes (such as generalization or composition) and learning strategies (such as elaboration or rehearsal). For instance, elaboration, analyzing incoming information in terms of existing knowledge, can be a conscious learning strategy. Although many do it automatically, and it is partially dependent upon the associative nature of memory, there is no reason it could not be taught and learned and improved through practice. Further, the contents and structure of the knowledge base determine how sucessfully particular information can be elaborated. To continue with our example from a previous section, a child who is just starting to learn about dinosaurs might only have one schema for encoding dinosaurs. For this novice child, learning about a meat-eating dinosaur with sharp teeth and a short neck probably requires the storage of the particular dinosaur name along with all this property information. For the expert child, however, who has many subschemas of different types of dinosaurs, the dinosaur's characteristics fit immediately into the slots of the meat-eater schema. The information that it is a meat eater is simply redundant confirmation that the right schema has been activated. This schema gives immediate access to examples of other meat-eaters, and the child can compare them with the new example in order to determine its discriminating characteristics and encode them. This example serves to point out how the declarative encoding process can vary as a function of existing knowledge structure. In this situation, because the expert child need not encode the basic features common to the meat-eater schema and has rapid access to other specific examples, a more sophisticated learning strategy may be employed. The novice child may also be able to compare examples and seek discriminating features but, in this case, the knowledge base does not allow it.

Thus, in a sense, learning to learn is definitely possible. However, it need not be basic learning processes that are learned or improved, but higher level strategies, and even in cases where similar strategies are available, the interaction of these strategies with the knowledge base is very important. A more complete knowledge base may allow more efficient learning without any differences at all in learning strategies and processes.

Acknowledgement

Preparation of this paper was supported in part by the Learning Research and Development Center, University of Pittsburgh, which is funded in part by the National Institute of Education (NIE). Further support was provided by the Spencer Foundation. The opinions expressed do not necessarily reflect the position or policy of the NIE or the Spencer Foundation and no official endorsement should be inferred. The authors would like to thank *Mary Beth Curtis* and *Robert Glaser* for their comments on earlier drafts of this paper.

References

Anderson, J.R.: Language, memory and thought (Erlbaum, Hillsdale 1976).

Anderson, J.R.: Acquisition of cognitive skill. Tech. Rep. 81–1 (Carnegie-Mellon University, Department of Psychology, Pittsburgh 1981).

Anderson, J.R.; Bower, G.H.: Human associative memory (Winston, Washington 1973).

Anderson, J.R.; Greeno, J.G.; Kline, P.J.; Neves, D.M.: Acquisition of problem-solving skill; in Anderson, Cognitive skills and their acquisition, pp. 191–230 (Erlbaum, Hillsdale 1981).

Bartlett, F.C.: Remembering: a study in experimental and social psychology (Cambridge University Press, Cambridge 1932).

Baylor, G.W.; Gascon, J.: An information processing theory of aspects of the development of weight seriation in children. Cognitive Psychol. *1:* 1–40 (1974).

Brown, A.L.: The development of memory: knowing, knowing about knowing, knowing how to know; in Reese, Advances in child development and behavior, vol. 10, pp. 104–152 (Academic Press, New York 1975).

Brown, A.L.: Learning and development: the problems of compatibility, access, and induction. Hum. Dev. *25:* 89–115 (1982).

Brown, A.L.; Campione, J.C.: Inducing flexible thinking: a problem of access; in Friedman, Das, O'Connor, Intelligence and learning, pp. 515–529 (Plenum Press, New York 1981).

Bruner, J.S.; Olver, R.R.; Greenfield, P.M.: Studies in cognitive growth (Wiley, New York 1966).

Carey, S.: Are children fundamentally different kinds of thinkers and learners than adults?; in Chipman, Segal, Glaser, Thinking and learning skills: current research and open questions, vol. 2 (Erlbaum, Hillsdale, in press).

Case, R.: Validation of a neo-Piagetian capacity construct. J. exp. Child Psychol. *14:* 287–302 (1972).

Chase, W.G.; Ericsson, K.A.: Skilled memory; in Anderson, Cognitive skills and their acquisition, pp. 141–189 (Erlbaum, Hillsdale 1981).

Chase, W.G.; Simon, H.A.: Perception in chess. Cognitive Psychol. *4:* 55–81 (1973a).

Chase, W.G.; Simon, H.A.: The mind's eye in chess; in Chase, Visual information processing (Academic Press, New York 1973b).

Chi, M.T.H.: Short-term memory limitations in children: capacity or processing deficits? Memory Cognition *4:* 559–572 (1976).

Chi, M.T.H.: Knowledge structures and memory development; in Siegler, Children's thinking: What develops?, pp. 73–96 (Erlbaum, Hillsdale 1978).

Chi, M.T.H.: Interactive roles of knowledge and strategies in the development of organized sorting and recall; in Chipman, Segal, Glaser, Thinking and learning skills: current research and open questions, vol. 2 (Erlbaum, Hillsdale, in press, a).

Chi, M.T.H.: Knowledge-derived categorization in young children; in Rogers, Sloboda, Acquisition of symbolic skills (Plenum Press, New York, in press, b).

Chi, M.T.H.; Koeske, R.D.: Network representation of a child's dinosaur knowledge. Devl. Psychol. *19:*29–39 (1983).

Childs, M.K.; Polich, J.M.: Developmental differences in mental rotation. J. exp. Child Psychol. *27:* 339–351 (1979).

Collins, A.; Loftus, E.F.: A spreading activation theory of semantic processing. Psychol. Rev. *82:* 407–428 (1975).

Collins, A.; Quillian, M.R.: Retrieval time from semantic memory. J. verb. Learn. verb. Behav. *8:* 240–247 (1969).

Cooper, L.A.; Shepard, R.N.: Chronometric studies of the rotation of mental images; in Chase, Visual information processing, pp. 75–176 (Academic Press, New York 1973).

Corsini, D.A.: Memory: interaction of stimulus and organismic factors. Hum. Dev. *14:* 227–235 (1971).

Dempster, F.M.: Memory span and short-term memory capacity: a developmental study. J. exp. Child Psychol. *26:* 419–431 (1978).

Ericsson, K.A.; Simon, H.A.: Verbal reports as data. Psychol. Rev. *87:* 215–253 (1980).

Fischer, K.W.: A theory of cognitive development: the control and construction of hierarchies of skills. Psychol. Rev. *87:* 477–531 (1980).

Flavell, J.H.: The developmental psychology of Jean Piaget (Van Nostrand, Princeton 1963).

Flavell, J.H.: Development studies of mediated memory; in Reese, Lipsitt, Advances in child development and behavior, vol. 5, pp. 182–211 (Academic Press, New York 1970).

Flavell, J.H.: First discussant's comments: What is memory development the development of? Hum. Dev. *14:* 272–278 (1971).

Flavell, J.H.: An analysis of cognitive developmental sequences. Genet. Psychol. Monogr. *86:* 279–350 (1972).

Gagné, R.M.: Contributions of learning to human development. Psychol. Rev. *75:* 177–191 (1968).

Gallagher, J.D.; Thomas, J.R.: Effects of varying post-KR intervals upon children's motor performance. J. Motor Behav. *12:* 41–56 (1980).

Gelman, R.: Conservation acquisition: a problem of learning to attend to relevant attributes. J. exp. Child Psychol. *7:* 167–187 (1969).

Gelman, R.: Cognitive development. A. Rev. Psychol. *29:* 297–332 (1978).

Gesell, A.: Infancy and human growth (Macmillan, New York 1928).

Gesell, A.; Thompson, H.: Learning and growth in identical twin infants. Genet. Psychol. Monogr. *6:* 1-24 (1929).

Halford, G.S.; Macdonald, C.: Children's pattern construction as a function of age and complexity. Child Dev. *48:* 1096–1100 (1977).

Halford, G.S.; Wilson, W.H.: A category theory approach to cognitive development. Cognitive Psychol. *12:* 356–411 (1980).

Hayes, J.R.; Simon, H.A.: Psychological differences among problem isomorphs; in Castellan, Pisoni, Potts, Cognitive theory, vol. 2, pp. 21–41 (Erlbaum, Hillsdale 1977).

Johnson-Laird, P.N.; Wason, P.C.: A theoretical analysis of insight into a reasoning task. Cognitive Psychol. *1:* 134–148 (1970).

Kail, R.V.; Hagen, J.W.: Perspectives on the development of memory and cognition (Erlbaum, Hillsdale 1977).

Kail, R.V.; Pellegrino, J.; Carter, P.: Developmental changes in mental rotation. J. exp. Child Psychol. *29:* 102–116 (1980).

Keil, F.C.: Constraints on knowledge and cognitive development. Psychol. Rev. *88:* 197–227 (1981).

Klahr, D.; Wallace, J.G.: Class inclusion processes; in Farnham-Diggory, Information processing in children, pp. 143–172 (Academic Press, New York 1972).

Kosslyn, S.D.: The representational-development hypothesis; in Ornstein, Memory development in children, pp. 157–189 (Erlbaum, Hillsdale 1978).

Langley, P.; Simon, H.A.: The central role of learning in cognition; in Anderson, Cognitive skills and their acquisition, pp. 361–380 (Erlbaum, Hillsdale 1981).

Lawler, R.W.: The progressive construction of mind. Cognitive Sci. *5:* 1–30 (1981).

Liben, L.S.: The developmental study of children's memory; in Field, Huston, Quay, Troll, Finly, Review of human development (Wiley, New York, in press).

Lindberg, M.A.: Is knowledge base development a necessary and sufficient condition for memory development? J. exp. Child Psychol. *30:* 401–410 (1980).

Mandler, G.: The construction and limitation of consciousness. Proc. Int. Symp. on Perspectives on Psychological Experimentation, Bad Homburg 1981.

Mandler, J.M.: Representation; in Flavell, Markman, Cognitive development, vol. 2 of Mussen, Carmichael's manual of child psychology (Wiley, New York, in press).

Marmor, G.S.: Development of kinetic images: When does the child first represent movement in mental images? Cognitive Psychol. *7:* 548–559 (1975).

McLaughlin, G.H.: Psycho-logic: a possible alternative to Piaget's formulation. Br. J. educ. Psychol. *33:* 61–67 (1963).

Miller, G.A.: The magical number seven plus or minus two: some limits on our capacity for processing information. Psychol. Rev. *63:* 81–97 (1956).

Minsky, M.A.: A framework for representing knowledge; in Winston, The psychology of computer vision (McGraw-Hill, New York 1975).

Nelson, K.: Semantic development and the development of semantic memory; in Nelson, Children's language, vol. 1, pp. 39–80 (Gardner Press, New York 1978).

Neves, D.M.; Anderson, J.R.: Knowledge compilation: mechanisms for the automatization of cognitive skills; in Anderson, Cognitive skills and their acquisition, pp. 57–84 (Erlbaum, Hillsdale 1981).

Newell, A.: Production systems: models of control structures; in Chase, Visual information processing, pp. 463–526 (Academic Press, New York 1973).

Newell, A.; Simon, H.A.: Human problem solving (Prentice Hall, Englewood Cliffs 1972).

Norman, D.A.: Notes toward a theory of complex learning; in Lesgold, Pellegrino, Fokkema, Glaser, Cognitive psychology and instruction (Plenum, New York 1978).

Norman, D.A.; Rumelhart, D.E.: Explorations in cognition (Freeman, San Francisco 1975).

Olson, G.M.: Developmental changes in memory and the acquisition of language; in Moore,

Cognitive development and the acquisition of language, pp. 145–157 (Academic Press, New York 1973).
Ornstein, P.A.: Memory development in children (Erlbaum, Hillsdale 1978).
Ornstein, P.A.; Naus, M.J.: Rehearsal processes in children's memory; in Ornstein, Memory development in children, pp. 69–99 (Erlbaum, Hillsdale 1978).
Paivio, A.: Imagery and verbal processes (Holt, New York 1971).
Pascual-Leone, J.: A mathematical model for the transition rule in Piaget's developmental stages. Acta psychol. *32:* 301–345 (1970).
Piaget, J.: Judgment and reasoning in the child (Harcourt, Brace & World, New York 1928).
Piaget, J.: The theory of stages in cognitive development; in Green, Ford, Flamer, Measurement and Piaget, pp. 1–11 (McGraw-Hill, New York 1971).
Piaget, J.: Intellectual evolution from adolescence to adulthood. Hum. Dev. *15:* 1–12 (1972).
Quillian, M.R.: Semantic memory (Bolt, Beranek & Newman, Cambridge 1966).
Riley, M.S.; Greeno, J.G.; Heller, J.I.: Development of children's problem-solving ability in arithmetic; in Ginsberg, The development of mathematical thinking (Academic Press, New York, in press).
Robertson, M.A.: Longitudinal evidence for developmental stages in the forceful overarm throw. J. Hum. Movmnt Stud. *4:* 167–175 (1978).
Rosch, E.; Lloyd, B.B.: Cognition and categorization (Erlbaum, Hillsdale 1978).
Rozin, P.: The evolution of intelligence and access to the cognitive unconscious; in Sprague, Epstein, Progress in psychobiology and physiological psychology, vol. 6, pp. 245–280 (Academic Press, New York 1976).
Rumelhart, D.E.; Lindsay, P.; Norman, D.A.: A process model for long-term memory; in Tulving, Donaldson, Organization of memory (Academic Press, New York, 1972).
Rumelhart, D.E.; Norman, D.A.: Accretion; tuning and restructuring: three modes of learning, Tech. Rep. CHIP 63 (University of California, San Diego Center for Human Information Processing, La Jolla 1976).
Rumelhart, D.E.; Norman, D.A.: Analogical processes in learning; in Anderson, Cognitive skills and their acquisition, pp. 335–359 (Erlbaum, Hillsdale 1981).
Rumelhart, D.E.; Norman, D.A.: Simulating a skilled typist: a study of cognitive-motor performance. Cognitive Sci. *6:* 1–36 (1982).
Rumelhart, D.E.; Ortony, A.: The representation of knowledge in memory; in Anderson, Spiro, Montague, Schooling and the acquisition of knowledge (Erlbaum, Hillsdale 1977).
Scardamalia, M.: Information processing capacity and the problem of horizontal decalage: a demonstration using combinatorial reasoning tasks. Child Dev. *48:* 28–37 (1977).
Schank, R.C.; Abelson, R.P.: Scripts, plans, goals and understanding: an inquiry into human knowledge structures (Erlbaum, Hillsdale 1977).
Siegler, R.S.: Three aspects of cognitive development. Cognitive Psychol. *8:* 481–520 (1976).
Siegler, R.S.: Developmental sequences within and between concepts. Soc. Res. Child Dev. Monogr. *46:* (1981).
Siegler, R.S.; Robinson, M.: The development of numerical understandings; in Reese, Lipsett, Advances in child development and behavior, vol. 16 (Academic Press, New York 1981).
Simon, H.A.: On the development of the processor; in Farnham-Diggory, Information processing in children, pp. 3–22 (Academic Press, New York 1972).
Simon, H.A.: How big is a chunk? Science *183:* 482–488 (1974).

Vuyk, R.: Overview and critique of Piaget's genetic epistemology (Academic Press, London 1981).

Waterman, D.A.: Adaptive production systems. Proc. 4th Int. Joint Conf. on Artificial Intelligence, pp. 296–303 (1975).

Young, R.M.: Strategies and the structure of a cognitive skill; in Underwood, Strategies of information processing, pp. 35–45 (Academic Press, London 1978).

Contr. hum. Dev., vol. 9, pp. 108–115 (Karger, Basel 1983)

Discussion: The Past Ten Years

Gary M. Olson

University of Michigan, Ann Arbor, Mich., USA

It is the evening of April 1, 1971. Professor Rip van Winkle has just listened to a symposium entitled 'What is Memory Development the Development of?' He is excited by what he has heard. After decades of neglect, the study of memory development in children has finally become a recognized field. Appropriately, the organizer of *that* symposium, *John Flavell*, has played a main role in initiating the study of memory development. A variety of interesting findings, concepts, and issues have been presented by the participants in that symposium. There is much excitement in the air, and *Jim Jenkins*, the second discussant captures this mood at the end of his discussion:

> 'The work you have heard tonight testifies to the vigor and the diversity of the research on the development of memory. The tenacity of pursuit and the ingenuity of the studies testifies to the high caliber of the talented people working in the field ... As we sail off into the sunset, I am happy to predict that this field is going to see explosive growth. I think that the new generation of researchers on the platform and in the audience tonight will assimilate and accommodate furiously to move the field to a new stage of deep understanding of the nature of cognitive memory' [*Jenkins*, 1971, p. 285].

Excited and eager, Professor van Winkle heads off to the bar to discuss the evening's proceedings with his friends. Later, enthused but exhausted, he heads off to his room for what he hopes will be a contented sleep before the next day's meeting. Indeed, it is a contented, but long, sleep. He falls into a deep slumber and awakens on April 2, but it is 1981 instead of 1971. He is confused, of course. He inquires as to what has happened to the meetings and is told that they are currently in session in Boston. So, slightly puzzled but nonetheless still eager, he heads off for Boston and by coincidence arrives just in time to hear tonight's symposium.

My role in these proceedings is to comment on what has happened over the past decade. I see this role as having two aspects, one narrow and one broad. The narrow task is to examine the two symposia for their similarities and contrasts. This is the past decade as viewed by our sleepy colleague, Professor van Winkle. How do tonight's contributions compare to those of 10 years ago?

The second and broader aspect of my role is to take a view that goes beyond the symposia and to look at the general field of memory development over the past 10 years. The two symposia contain important samples of work from their respective periods, but also miss much, and merely looking at their contents does not capture all of what has gone on in the past decade.

Both my narrow and my broad survey of the past decade will have the general theme that both a lot has happened and too little has happened. Professor van Winkle would notice a lot of *change*, but the deeper question is, would he observe a lot of *progress*?

Let's turn to the narrow task first. What would Professor van Winkle's perceptions be of this evening's symposium? Clearly, he would have to be impressed with the new set of faces. Though there are some exceptions, most of the participants entered the memory development scene sometime during the 1970s, in many cases as graduate students. Professor van Winkle would be encouraged by this. New blood is generally a symptom of a field with continuing life. After a decade, the second, third, and perhaps even fourth generation of memory development researchers are among us. The field is very much alive.

Professor van Winkle would also notice a shift of some kind in the conceptual framework. The 1971 symposium showed a strong influence of the information-processing psychology of the late 1960s. What *Klatzky* [1975] has called the modal model of memory, best exemplified by *Atkinson and Shiffrin* [1968], was evident in a number of the 1971 presentations. This reflected some general trends in the psychology of memory during that period. The late 1960s saw the flowering of the field of memory in psychology after a long period of misdirection, confusion, and sterility. A rich array of new data and theory emerged that was bound to influence the developmental study of memory. The 1971 symposium certainly reflected the general zeitgeist of the cognitive psychology of its era.

Professor van Winkle would find the present symposium less coherent in this regard. He would notice a shift away from the theoretical concepts so central in 1971 but, despite a lot of new vocabulary, he would have a hard time seeing a clear alternative theoretical formulation underlying tonight's talks. This puzzled reaction would be the right one. The study of memory in general and memory development in particular has lost what was probably only the illusion of theoretical coherence that it seemed to have in 1971. For the most part, research has focused on particular phenomena, with no general theory emerging that has gained wide acceptance. Professor van Winkle would not understand the passing references of tonight's participants to levels of processing or ACT, but he would accurately perceive that these theories have not generally taken hold.

Having heard *Flavell* [1971] use the term metamemory at the close of his discussion in 1971, Professor van Winkle would be extremely interested to find a whole paper devoted to this topic in 1981. And he would be struck by two things: the stress that *Henry Wellman* placed on definitional issues, and the generally apologetic tone of his discussion. Professor van Winkle would rightly conclude that here seems to be a concept that has enjoyed a lot of popularity but has recently been subjected to a lot of criticism. He should be grateful to *Henry* for so clearly setting forth the key issues. There has been an inordinate amount of confusion about what the term metamemory means, and this has led many to conclude that it is merely a new, misleading name for old familiar concepts or else is an elusive, vague concept. *Henry's* table I shows quite clearly the multiple phenomena that have come to be associated with this concept. His attempt to clarify what is meant is an essential step. That he was forced to do this is indicative of the meta-mess many have found themselves in when trying to understand this work.

The apologetic tone is also revealing. The idea behind the study of metamemory is that one of the things a child learns is something about the nature of his own mind. I very much like *Henry's* description of this as the child's theory of mind. Presumably this knowledge is important to the study of development because this knowledge ought to come to play a role in memory performance or in the development of memory skills. *Henry* is forced to be apologetic because the evidence has not been very good on this. To his credit, *Henry* provides a sophisticated analysis of why null results might have arisen, and then presents some important non-null results. But Professor van Winkle would be quite curious. Maybe there is no connection between metamemory knowledge and memory development? The case is still open.

I have always been puzzled by the insularity of metamemory research. It has primarily been confined to development psychology. Though there are bits and pieces of such work in the adult literature, it is not an idea which has caught on more generally. I think *Henry* has eloquently captured why it hasn't: The concept isn't clear enough, and both the theoretical and empirical issue of its connections to memory performance is too uncertain. To edge into *Tom Trabasso's* turf for a moment, Professor van Winkle might well wonder whether we'll be revisiting metamemory in 1991.

The presentation which would seem most familiar to Professor van Winkle was by *Naus and Ornstein*. The issues raised there have the greatest continuity with the issues raised in 1971. The participants of 10 years ago pretty well agreed that one of the things that develops in memory is the availability and use of strategies. Thus, research on this topic was seen then and is still seen now as at the core of the study of memory development. While *Naus and Ornstein* described a variety of work on strategies, their newer work on the relationship between strategies and knowledge is sure to be an important line of work. Strategy development is unlikely to have a monolithic role in memory development.

The discussion of strategies played a large role in the 1971 symposium, but in his discussion *Flavell* [1971] pointed out his and others' uneasiness at the elusiveness of this concept. Has our understanding of what strategies are and how they appear in development substantially advanced during the past decade? I wonder if Professor van Winkle could be convinced.

The topics addressed by *Nelson* and by *Chi and Rees* would be exceptionally interesting to Professor van Winkle. These papers most clearly reflect new developments since 1971, and he would clearly agree with the importance both papers give to the acquisition of knowledge in the development of memory. The governing intuition would strike him as obvious: What a child knows about a topic should affect his or her ability to learn and remember material on that topic. Both papers subscribe to this view and even flirt with the strong position that development may be little more than the acquisition of knowledge. Neither quite adopts this strong view, but the enormous importance both place on knowledge acquisition is a stark contrast with the discussion of 10 years ago.

He would not be acquainted with the concept of a script, not knowing the work of *Schank and Abelson* [1977] on this particular representation. He would not know what to make of the concept. What is the status of script theory as a psychological theory? What alternatives exist? How does the research of *Nelson* and others either affirm or disconfirm the script theory? He would not be familiar with any of the theories of knowledge representation that have been stimulated by work in artificial intelligence, but would note that a whole new theoretical vocabulary has been introduced into psychology.

Another feature of *Nelson's* work would be striking. Much of what she is examining is the natural world knowledge of children: what they know about the objects and events of their everyday life. Her research has used interview and other techniques to more exactly describe this knowledge. This represents an important trend in current work on memory development and *Nelson* is only one of several investigators who are attempting to focus on the child's world. He would undoubtedly be pleased with this trend.

The *Chi and Rees* paper reviews a number of positions and issues pertaining to memory development and the role of knowledge acquisition in it. The demonstrations that knowledgeable kids can do better than unknowledgeable adults is interesting and important, and *Chi and Rees* are correct in citing the challenge this finding provides for several major views of memory development. This paper is important in attempting to go beyond the mere suggestion that there is a strong link between expertise and development. A number of factors that could be involved in memory development are described, and an attempt is made to link the role of knowledge acquisition to an amalgam of two important theories of the 1970s. But there are still some important clarifications that need to be made. What are the differences between experts and novices, adults and kids, bright and dull? In general, the first member of each of these pairs knows more than the second. But it seems fairly obvious that despite this homology there are strong differences between each of these pairs too. A clearer understanding of such differences should help clarify the role of knowledge acquisition in memory development.

Now I'd like to turn my attention to the broader view and my mechanism for doing this will be to present a short list of phenomena or issues studied during the 1970s that did not appear in tonight's symposium. The reason for doing this is to convince Professor van Winkle that one of the hallmarks of the past decade is the quantity and diversity of research on this topic. My list is idiosyncratic and incomplete, but hopefully it is suggestive. So, in no particular order, here are some of the other topics that could have appeared in tonight's symposium.

Infant Memory. If Professor van Winkle were to look through the 1981 Society for Research in Child Development (SRCD) program he would have to be struck with the quantity and diversity of infant research going on today. The 1970s have certainly been the decade of the infant in developmental psychology and, happily, the study of learning and memory in infants flourished during this period. The study of infant habituation and its variants has been widespread, and by any metric our understanding of the infant's ability to learn and remember has undergone marked advances [*Olson and Sherman*, in press]. However, I don't want to mislead you, Professor van Winkle. There is still a huge gap between what we would like to know and what we do know, but any general theory of memory development will need to take account of where the child starts out and research on infant learning and memory is beginning to provide some hints of this.

Memory in Preschoolers. Research on children in the preschool period has always been limited, but during the late 1970s several clever investigators, including *Henry Wellman* and *Katherine Nelson*, came up with a variety of techniques, based on the naturally occurring behavior of preschoolers, to study their learning and retention. Once again, there is not yet a lot to say about this work, but along with the work on infancy it will provide needed information about the appearance of memory skill prior to school. All too often the preschool child has been the developmental foil, the child who lacks what the older child possesses. Thankfully, this view is changing. We are beginning to learn what the preschooler is like, rather than what he or she is not like.

School Learning. Several of tonight's papers presented research on the role of real world knowledge on learning and memory and this represents a general, healthy trend in the 1970s. It has had other manifestations. For instance, there has been much research on learning and memory of textual materials, especially stories. In general, cognitive psychology has been much more interested in memory for classroom or everyday materials. Professor van Winkle would have to feel some sense of appropriateness in this, even if the payoff for this shift is yet to come.

Cross-Cultural Research. Throughout the 1970s a variety of investigators examined learning and memory phenomena in children in a variety of cultures. Often this work attempted to address the important theoretical questions of the role of schooling in cognitive development. Given the complexity of carrying out and interpreting cross-cultural investigations it is probably too soon to reach firm, general conclusions, but this type of research will provide an important source of knowledge about the nature of memory development.

Possible Structural Limits on Memory. There was a flurry of activity during the mid to late 1970s on the question of why measured memory span changes with age [*Chi*, 1976, 1977; *Huttenlocher and Burke*, 1976; *Olson*, 1973; *Simon*, 1974]. At issue was the nature of the development of one of the most fundamental limitations on human cognition, namely the limited ability to hold more than a handful of items of information actively in mind at once. The developmental question is interesting because it raises so many fundamental issues: the nature of chunking, strategies, memory for order, encoding speed, rehearsal, the organization of output, etc. There is no firm resolution to the question of why memory span increases with age, but one cannot help but believe that many key insights into the nature of memory development will come from the analysis of this specific question.

Piaget. The English translation of *Memory and Intelligence* appeared in 1973, and *Piaget and Inhelder's* [1973] idea that memory may improve between the initial experience and later retention because of increased understanding of the original phenomena attracted a lot of attention. Much American work has called this phenomenon or its interpretation into question [reviews by *Liben*, 1977a, b], but the idea certainly represents an interesting challenge to the thinking of memory development researchers.

The Renewal of the Study of Intelligence. During the 1970s there was renewed interest in intelligence and its components. While concepts like induction or analogical thinking are obviously key components of intelligence, memory factors also play a large role, and the study of memory development in relation to intelligence in general is a useful departure.

Well, Professor van Winkle, it has been an active decade. You cannot help but be impressed by the amount of activity. But has there been progress? Certainly there has been change, and new topics not central in 1971 have received extensive investigation. The 1971 symposium was quite thorough in raising candidate answers in response to the question: 'What is memory development the development of?' Tonight's panel might rank order these answers somewhat differently than the group 10 years ago, the role of knowledge being the clearest example. However, we still lack a *general* account of what memory *development* is. There is still a lot of work left to do.

References

Atkinson, R.C.; Shiffrin, R.M.: Human memory: a proposed system and its control processes; in Spence, Spence, The psychology of learning and motivation, vol. 2, pp. 328–372 (Academic Press, New York 1968).

Chi, M.T.H.: Short-term memory limitations in children: capacity or processing deficits? Memory Cognition *4:* 559–572 (1976).

Chi, M.T.H.: Age differences in memory span. J. exp. Child Psychol. *23:* 266–281 (1977).

Flavell, J.H.: First discussant's comments: What is memory development the development of? Hum. Dev. *14:* 272–278 (1971).

Huttenlocher, J.; Burke, D.: Why does memory span increase with age? Cognitive Psychol. *8:* 1–31 (1976).

Jenkins, J.J.: Second discussant's comments: What's left to say? Hum. Dev. *14:* 279–286 (1971).

Klatzky, R.L.: Human memory: structure and processes (Freeman, San Francisco 1975).

Liben, L.S.: Memory from a cognitive-developmental perspective: a theoretical and empirical review; in Overton, Gallagher, Knowledge and development, vol. 1, pp. 149–203 (Plenum Press, New York 1977a).

Liben, L.S.: Memory in the context of cognitive development: the Piagetian approach; in Kail, Hagen, Perspectives on the development of memory and cognition, pp. 297–331 (Erlbaum, Hillsdale 1977b).

Olson, G.M.: Developmental changes in memory and the acquisition of language; in Moore, Cognitive development and the acquisition of language, pp. 145–157 (Academic Press, New York 1973).

Olson, G.M.; Sherman, T.: Attention, learning, and memory in infants; in Haith, Campos, Manual of child psychology, vol. 2 (Wiley, New York, in press).

Piaget, J.; Inhelder, B.: Memory and intelligence (Routledge & Kegan Paul, London 1973).

Schank, R.C.; Abelson, R.: Scripts, plans, goals, and understanding (Erlbaum, Hillsdale 1977).

Simon, H.A.: How big is a chunk? Science *183:* 482–488 (1974).

Contr. hum. Dev., vol. 9, pp. 116–122 (Karger, Basel 1983)

Discussion: What Is Memory Development To Be the Development of?

Tom Trabasso [1]

University of Chicago, Chicago, Ill., USA

It is an honor to discuss memory and its development in a symposium which marks the 10th anniversary of the one organized by *John Flavell*. My duty, as reflected in the title borrowed from *Flavell* and modified by me, is to serve as a prognosticator and anticipate another symposium in the year 1991, marking the 20th anniversary of the *Flavell* symposium and the 10th anniversary of the *Chi* symposium. Note that it is possible to accumulate in this manner anniversaries at the rate of one per decade for as long as interest in memory and its development continues. In addition, *Gary Olson's* professor, Rip van Winkle, would have to be programmed to have a regular sleep-wake cycle of 10-year periods in order to express his surprise at what happened retrospectively.

Predicting the future follows a variant of Murphy's law: whatever can be predicted will go wrong. At least my prognostication can serve as a contrastive point of departure for future *Gary Olsons*, should the 1991 symposium on memory development occur. With these expectations in mind, I accept my responsibility as seer and project into the decade ahead.

When we predict the future, we frequently make linear extrapolations of the present. Thus, one expectation is that *Flavell's* original question will continue to be a central one: 'What is memory development the development of?' In answer and in anticipating what may occur as answers, there are two interpretations of this question which deserve examination. First, we ask, 'What is memory?' and second, 'How does memory develop?'

A safe prediction is that the main question and its component interpretation will continue to guide and dominate research on memory development. However, while the question remains the same, the answers will

[1] The writing of this paper was supported by National Institute of Education Grant NIE-G-79-0125.

change. The reason is that our conceptions of both memory and development lack permanence and undergo transformations of meaning despite the efforts of researchers, editors, textbook writers and other professionals to conserve them.

In 1971, the conception of memory was largely one of an 'outside-in' or 'bottom-up' process. Information was received from the environment as a stimulus input, held in various, successive and temporary stores until, through recoding and other transformations, it reached a more or less permanent store. Control mechanisms such as rehearsal, grouping, chunking and organizing were performed while the information resided in an intermediate store known as short-term memory. The final resting place, called long-term memory, had, in this conceptualization, a small effect on what occurred during encoding and subsequent storage or retrieval. As *Naus and Ornstein* have pointed out in the present symposium, this model of the 1960s guided the research that followed in the 1970s either explicitly or implicitly. Research on strategies and metamemory (control or executive processes), discussed respectively by *Naus and Ornstein* and by *Wellman*, became of central concern when children rather than adult human beings were the subjects of study. Memory development, then, was the study of the emergence, acquisition or manifestation of strategies or strategic knowledge (procedures or procedural knowledge). Knowing *how to* use mnemonic operations and knowing *about* these operations and their effects on data received from the task environment fascinated those of us in the memory game.

The answer to the question of what is memory, however, underwent a shift. The 'outside-in' or the 'bottom-up', multi-storage memory models were turned on their sides or their heads and became 'inside-out' or 'top-down' and centered on *knowledge*. What the child knows as he or she moves from novice to expert determines what he or she attends to, encodes, stores and retrieves. *Nelson, Wellman, Chi* and *Rees* each and collectively reflect this conceptually driven view of memory and its development.

What then is memory development? Early on, it was the expansion of memory capacity or space via use of procedural knowledge. Later, it was the expansion of a knowledge base over successive, specific domains.

What, then, is memory development *to be* the development of? We shall probably continue to believe that children and adults have limitations on how much information they can pay attention to, encode, store and retrieve. Memory development is, then, the increase in these capacities or a decrease in the limitations. If we view information processing as the allocation by the child of his or her resources to the problem at hand, then limitations of processing can occur for three reasons: (1) limitations on resources, (2) limitations on resource allocation, and (3) limitations in the data constrained by the environment. An interaction between these sources – the task environment, the resources available and the child's control over resource allocation – appears to summarize, in different terminology and metaphors, an emerging view expressed in the present symposium and augers the future.

The recent emphasis on knowledge, stimulated by the use of knowledge bases in process models by workers in artificial intelligence, stresses the importance of the resources the child has to bring to bear upon the task. These resources include not only declarative and procedural knowledge (content and memory operations) but also structured knowledge or schemas such as *Nelson* has assumed to be used in her studies on the development of scripts.

Given a changing knowledge base, the child also has to learn ways in which these resources can be allocated to the task at hand, criteria for the selection of appropriate resources and that sustained or repeated efforts are necessary for successful allocation. This kind of executive control and decision-making reflects developing goals or motivational systems in the child as well as metacognitive components which are more knowledge based.

Turning to the environment, we need to look at how these things change with development and assess what kind of data is presented to the child for encoding, storing and retrieving. In short, we ask: What is required of the child? Is it encoding? If so, to what extent? Is it retrieval? If so, how much and what kind? Does the child have to identify, reconstruct or recall something? Then, we ask, what are the data and how complex are they?

Surely, these factors operate interactively. For example, in *Wellman's* examination of organizational demands and the child's knowledge of organization, the interaction of these factors determines whether or not the child's performance is affected by his or her metacognitive resources. If the data complexity is low, then performance may be good, regardless of the amount of procedural knowledge the child has available – too few resources are required. If the demands are high (the data are complex or degraded) and exceed the child's resources, performance is poor, regardless of the amount of procedural knowledge available.

Consider children's comprehension of events such as scripts or stories. If the events lend themselves to a coherent interpretation based upon the child's knowledge of human intentionality and causation, then the data demands are low. If, however, the successive events are not causally related or connecting events are missing, then more effort at allocation and more resources are required. The child has to create different successive causal fields, infer missing events or connect remote ones in order to arrive at a coherent interpretation of the data. These additional demands cost time as well as effort and result in more limited representation of the data and poorer subsequent recall.

Memory development, then, appears to be the development of resources for different, successive domains of increasing complexity. The resources may, however, be knowledge that is both domain specific and domain independent. As the child enters into novel physical and social domains, he or she acquires both specific and general knowledge. The child's psychological movement through these physical and social domains places upon him or her different kinds of demands. Learning the domain leads to the acquisition of knowledge specific to it and interaction with the domain leads to better resource selection, planning, monitoring and allocation. Expertise is acquired within domains and the expert adult is one who has mastered a range of domains. In this view, the child is not viewed as lacking in knowledge. The child is viewed as acquiring the knowledge necessary to the domain in which he or she finds him or herself much like the adult who changes a job or enters into a new personal relationship with another adult. The child is becoming expert, achieving partial knowledge, and is increasingly successful in the domains in which he or she finds him or herself.

The future research on memory development might address the interplay of the child's domain (rather than the adult's domain as a frame of reference) with what the child knows and chart the development of that knowledge (and hence, memory skill) over the domain. This requires knowing what is the task and what does the child know about the task at the point in time the child is studied relative to the domain specified rather than to an adult normative reference.

The future research on memory development might also address the question of *acquisition* as well as the *retention* of knowledge. This latter assesses what is already known while the former determines how the knowledge is learned as well as what is learned. If we assume that knowledge is represented, we need to find out what is the nature of these representations and *how* they are constructed, modified or changed. The future research on memory development might focus on a problem-solving approach to both learning and memory. Learning here will not resemble necessarily the construction of associative networks. Rather, the focus might be on mechanisms for extracting or creating rules, productions and actions on structured domains and how these are organized into systems. In assessment, the future research on memory development might chart the knowledge base at times t and $t + k$, determining procedural and declarative changes over the k units in time. Further, if an event in the relevant domain occurs between t and $t + k$, then the change in the knowledge base as a result of a learning experience intervention may be determined.

The future research on memory development might address the question of demands the different domains make *on* or *for* memory. That is, when do occasions and opportunities for the use of memory begin or occur and in which domains are they most critical. A prime candidate is formal instruction and schooling. The school curriculum itself may be a rich source of the kinds and changes in demands for storage and retrieval of information. When do these demands begin, how often do they occur and to what extent do they give rise to procedures which are domain independent? These school domains may affect the executive processes and their acquisition as well. Are the curriculum and its tasks structured in such a way that children can acquire efficient procedures for using their resources? Is there evidence that teachers teach or model procedures? In short, what are the sources of our procedural and metacognitive knowledge?

The future research on memory development might examine more carefully the implications of theories about domain specific knowledge. The representation of knowledge in different domains may become a subject for study in its own right. This would mean analyses, discoveries and process modeling of memory operations in particular contexts. For example, in a closed domain such as chess, the representation of knowledge may be defined in terms of a set of basic procedures appropriate to a given level of expertise and performance. For example, the child knows the names of the pieces, their functions and their permissible moves but has not played many games. Another level would involve structures for opening, middle and end games. These and more advanced levels might involve representations or programs of goals and actions one takes given the conditions of the pieces in relation to one another at a given point of the game.

The future research on memory development might have to decide *which domains* are most significant to development and in what sequence they occur. A knowledge base approach would seem to require an answer to the question, which knowledge? Further, which domains and what experiences within them give rise to transfer of procedural knowledge across domains? One candidate for this is the domain of language, since language use in encoding and retrieval appears to be critical. However, the conceptual basis for language itself is largely unknown. If the novice-expert metaphor is to be of use, then the sequence of possible knowledge bases the child has as he or she develops from a novice to an intermediate to an expert will have to be traced both for particular domains such as mathematics and across domains such as social interaction. In the near future, development with restricted domains appears more likely to become the focus of inquiry.

The future research on memory development is likely to be plagued by related and persistent problems. In addition to deciding which domains are of developmental importance, how does a succession of domains actually characterize development? Are the domains overlapping or sequential? If domains interact, the questions of learning and transfer arise. In the case of language cited above, language qua language and its mnemonic functions may be domain-independent once acquired but the lexical items and their corresponding concepts may be domain particular. However, procedural knowledge expressed as mnemonic strategies may or may not be domain specific. The discovery and use of rehearsal and some organizational strategies seems to depend upon the use of tasks that involve unrelated materials, as *Naus and Ornstein* have mentioned. These strategies may be unnecessary for the comprehension and memory of connected discourse such as narratives. For example, the recall of stories does not show the serial position effects characteristic of word lists. Recall of events in stories would seem to be better understood in terms of the child's knowledge about human goals, plans, actions and outcomes.

Finally, the future research on memory development might address the persistent and nagging problem of individual differences. Will it suffice to describe individual differences in memory in terms of differences in the knowledge base? If so, what kinds of differences? How would such a position deal with the fact that individuals differ in the *rate* at which they seem to acquire the knowledge base as well as its composition?

In 1991, I hope that I have the privilege of attending a symposium on memory development held at the meetings of the Society for Research in

Child Development in order to hear what happened to the study of memory development in the 1980s. Perhaps I will be spared the embarrassment of serving as a straw person or a dead horse for flogging since there may not be such a symposium after all. Memory may, by that time, have lost its separate status as a psychological faculty and become a part of human cognition. If so, then the question won't be posed the way *John Flavell* did in 1971. The answer may finally have done away with the question.

Author Index

Subject Index